Evaluation
Nutshell

Evaluation
in a Nutshell

A practical
guide to the
evaluation
of health
promotion
programs

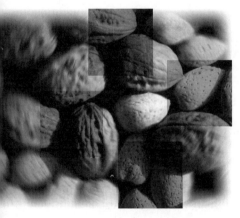

Don Nutbeam
Adrian Bauman

The McGraw·Hill Companies

Sydney New York San Francisco Auckland
Bangkok Bogotá Caracas Hong Kong
Kuala Lumpur Lisbon London Madrid
Mexico City Milan New Delhi San Juan
Seoul Singapore Taipei Toronto

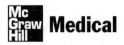 **Medical**

National Library of Australia Cataloguing-in-Publication data:

Nutbeam, Don.
Evaluating health promotion in a nutshell.
Includes index.

ISBN 0 074 71553 4.

1. Health promotion. 2. Health planning. I. Bauman, Adrian E. (Adrian Ernest). II. Title.
613

Published in Australia by
McGraw-Hill Australia Pty Ltd
Level 2, 82 Waterloo Road, North Ryde NSW 2113
Publisher: Nicole Meehan
Production Editor: Kathryn Murphy
Editor: Ruth Matheson
Proofreader: Tim Learner
Indexer: Glenda Browne
Designer (cover and interior): Jan Schmoeger, Designpoint
Illustrator: Alan Laver, Shelly Communications
Typeset in 10/12 pt ITC Giovanni Book by Jan Schmoeger, Designpoint
Printed on 80 gsm woodfree by 1010 Printing International Ltd, China.

Contents

Preface

This is a book for students of health promotion, and for health promotion practitioners. *Evaluation in a Nutshell* is intended to equip the reader with the ability to understand, interpret and assess the quality of published research, to excite interest in evaluation and promote further study that would lead to the development of core skills in evaluation. It provides foundation knowledge and recommended further reading.

In writing this book we have drawn upon many years of experience in teaching public health students, in conducting evaluations of health promotion programs and in working with health promotion practitioners. From this experience we have recognised the need for students and practitioners to understand the basic principles of evaluation, and the application of these principles in evaluation design—whether for the purposes of conducting an evaluation or assessing the published work of others.

Any review of published research will reveal that not all health promotion programs are equally successful in achieving their goals and objectives. Experience tells us that programs are most likely to be successful when the determinants of a health problem are well understood, where the needs and motivations of the target population are addressed, and the context in which the program is being implemented has been taken into account. That is, the program 'fits' the problem.

Similarly, in developing an evaluation design for a health promotion program, the evaluation design needs to fit the circumstances of the program. Not all programs need to be evaluated in the same ways, or with the same level of resources, or using the same evaluation designs. This book illustrates the ways in which evaluation questions change with the evolution of a program. It shows how those programs that are truly innovative, testing for the first time a potentially costly, controversial, or otherwise risky form of intervention, need close scrutiny and the most structured and comprehensive evaluation. On the other hand, programs that have previously been shown to work in a variety of circumstances, and are low cost and low risk, will require more modest monitoring for the purposes of accountability and quality control.

Evaluations have to be tailored to suit the activity and circumstances of individual programs—no single method or design can be 'right' for all programs.

Evaluation in a Nutshell provides an introduction to the strategic and technical issues in evaluation, and some of the practical and scientific challenges related to the evaluation of health promotion programs. The book takes a real public health focus. It not only includes individual interventions, but also considers how to influence whole communities or populations. Even for experienced researchers and practitioners, the book will provide a useful prompt on key issues, as well as guidance on how to organise and conduct evaluation studies.

Acknowledgments

Several people have contributed to the development of *Evaluation in a Nutshell*. We would like to acknowledge the contribution of Bill Bellew, Lesley King and Bill Reger-Nash for their constructive comments and advice on early drafts of the book.

Introduction

Evaluation is the formal process of judging the 'value' of some-thing. In health promotion, an evaluation will determine the extent to which a program has achieved its desired health outcomes, and will assess the contribution of the different processes that are used to achieve these outcomes. Scientists, health practitioners, politicians and the wider community all have different views on what represents 'value' from a health promotion program, how success should be defined and what should be measured. For example:

- Policy makers and budget managers need to judge the likely success of programs in order to make decisions about how to allocate resources, and to be accountable for these decisions. Success is often defined by the relationship between financial investment and the achievement of health outcomes in the short term.
- Health practitioners need to judge the likely and actual success of a program in achieving its defined health outcomes in 'real-life' situations, so that they know that their work is effective, and understand what needs to be done to ensure successful implementation. Success may be defined in terms of the effectiveness of the program in achieving health outcomes, the practicality of implementation, program sustainability and the maintenance of health gains in the longer term.
- The community who are to benefit from health promotion action may place great value on the processes through which a program is conducted, particularly whether or not the program is participatory and addresses priorities that the community itself has identified. Success may be defined in terms of relevance to perceived needs and opportunities for community participation.

- Academic researchers need to judge a program's success (or failure) in order to contribute to the science of health promotion and improve health promotion practice. Success may be defined in terms of the effects identified through rigorous study designs and measured through quantifiable and validated outcomes, and where the expected effects are theoretically based.

These perspectives are distinct, but not mutually exclusive. In each perspective success is judged through improved health outcomes, yet each differs greatly in the emphasis given to the cost, practicality and processes involved in achieving these outcomes. Correspondingly, there is a vast spectrum of approaches used to evaluate health promotion programs. These range from highly structured, methodology-driven evaluations that focus strongly on the measurement of outcomes, through to much less rigid, highly participatory forms of evaluation.

As practitioners, we need to be accountable for what we do, and we need to make explicit what we expect to achieve through the investments that are made in health promotion interventions. All programs can benefit from some form of evaluation, but not all require the same intensity of evaluation, or use the same criteria for success. Innovative programs using a costly or controversial intervention for the first time need close scrutiny with comprehensive evaluation. By contrast, programs that have been proven to work, are low-cost and uncontroversial require minimal monitoring for the purposes of accountability.

This book aims to:

- provide an overview and a simple classification system for the evaluation of a health promotion program;
- distinguish between formative, process, impact and outcome evaluation;
- consider the relative strengths of qualitative and quantitative research methods;
- provide practical guidance on when and how to evaluate programs, and the range of evaluation designs and research methods that can be used;
- consider how best to 'measure' health promotion activity and outcomes;
- provide a practical 'glossary' of terms used in health promotion program evaluation; and
- refer the reader to sources of further information.

Chapter 1
Planning for evaluation

It is best to consider evaluation during the planning stage as an integral part of the program. It is far more difficult to add the evaluation in at later stages—after all the critical decisions on program design and execution have been made.

Successful evaluation of a program is more likely if:

- a thorough analysis of the health problem is conducted to indicate the scope for intervention;
- there are clearly defined, logical and feasible program goals and objectives;
- formative assessment is used to develop an intervention, giving sufficient attention to the materials, resources and human capacity required for successful implementation;
- the program is implemented as planned;
- the program is of sufficient size, duration and sophistication to be proven effective or ineffective;
- there is clear direction on how the evaluation is to be conducted and what is to be measured; and
- the evaluation provides sufficient, relevant information to those who will decide the program's value.

Achieving these conditions for successful evaluation is challenging, but more likely if a structured approach to planning has been adopted.

Figure 1.1 presents a health promotion planning and evaluation cycle used in the companion book, *Theory in a Nutshell: A Practical Guide to Health Promotion Theories*. It indicates the various stages in the planning, implementation and evaluation of a health promotion program in the form of a cycle. Each of these stages is considered in turn.

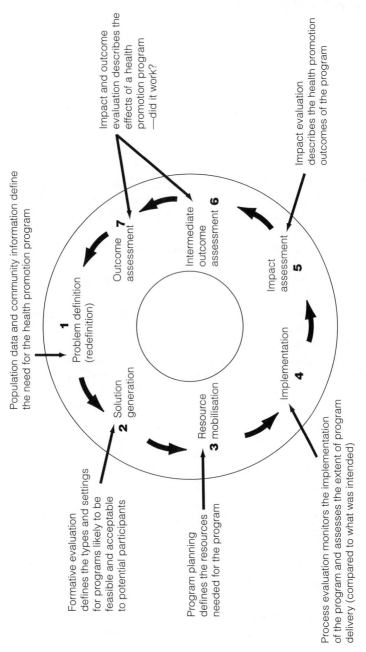

Population data and community information define the need for the health promotion program

Formative evaluation defines the types and settings for programs likely to be feasible and acceptable to potential participants

Program planning defines the resources needed for the program

Process evaluation monitors the implementation of the program and assesses the extent of program delivery (compared to what was intended)

Impact and outcome evaluation describes the effects of a health promotion program —did it work?

Impact evaluation describes the health promotion outcomes of the program

1 Problem definition (redefinition)

2 Solution generation

3 Resource mobilisation

4 Implementation

5 Impact assessment

6 Intermediate outcome assessment

7 Outcome assessment

Figure 1.1 Health promotion planning and evaluation cycle

Problem definition: starting at the end

A wide range of knowledge and information is gathered from various fields (e.g. epidemiology, demography, behavioural and social sciences) and, together with an understanding of community needs and priorities, is used to define a given health problem and generate potentially effective solutions. At this stage, it is important to take account of:

- the **prevalence** of the problem (the number of people affected) and whether the prevalence is different in various subgroups (such as older adults, adolescents, people from socially or culturally diverse groups);
- the public health impact of the problem (the seriousness of the consequences of the problem for the individuals affected and the population as a whole); and
- the potential for intervention (whether some factors that will have an impact on the problem can be changed, and the scale of the health improvement that could be achieved if the problem were reduced or abolished).

The analysis of this evidence should then lead to the development of measurable health promotion program goals and objectives that form the basis for the program plan. These are defined in Box 1.1.

Box 1.1 Health promotion program goals and objectives

Health promotion program **goals** are measurable changes in behaviours (e.g. smoking, food choices), or social, economic and environmental conditions (e.g. restrictions on smoking; food supply and promotion), which are the major determinants of the health outcomes (such as reduced heart disease or diabetes) that are being targeted. Program goals are an important **intermediate health outcome** of health promotion programs.

Health promotion program **objectives** are measurable changes to modifiable personal attributes (such as knowledge, motivations, skills), social norms and social support, and organisational factors (e.g. rules and processes) that influence the program goals. These measure the short-term outcomes of health promotion programs.

In this way, the beginning of the planning process is firmly focused on the end evaluation of outcomes through a thorough and logical analysis of the linkages between intervention and outcome. This phase ensures that there is a clear definition of who or what is the target of the intervention (subpopulation group, environmental or organisational element), and what outcomes will be sought. The early definition of these outcomes, and consideration of how they might be measured, is an important first stage in the evaluation process. The selection of outcome measures is described further in Chapter 5.

Solution generation

The second stage in the cycle—solution generation—indicates the need for the analysis of potential solutions, leading to the development of a **program plan**[1] that specifies the interventions to be employed, as well as the sequence of activity. This stage in the process indicates how and when change might be achieved in the target variable (population, organisation or policy). The processes of change within the program are identified, leading to the selection of effective interventions to achieve change and the timing and sequencing of interventions in order to achieve maximum effect.

A comprehensive health promotion program might consist of multiple interventions targeted at achieving different health promotion outcomes. Figure 1.2 provides an overview of the relationship between the 'process' of health promotion—described in the model as health promotion actions—and the different types of impact and outcome that such interventions might produce.

Working from the endpoint on the right-hand side of the model in Figure 1.2, *social and health outcomes* reflect a functional definition of health as the endpoint of health and medical interventions. Thus, outcomes such as quality of life, functional independence and equity have the highest value in the model. Related to this, though not the only influential factor, are health outcomes that can be more narrowly defined in terms of disease experience, physical and mental health status.

Intermediate health outcomes represent the *determinants* of the health and social outcomes. These include personal behaviours that provide protection from disease or injury (such as physical activity), or increased risk of ill-health (such as tobacco use),

---

[1] Words appearing in bold are included in the glossary on pp. 114–21.

Health promotion actions	Health promotion outcomes (outcomes of the process of intervention)	Intermediate health outcomes (program impact, or short-term outcomes)	Social health outcomes (long-term outcomes)
Education Examples include patient education, school education and broadcast media communication	*Health literacy* Measures include health-related knowledge, attitude, motivation, behavioural intentions, personal skills and self-efficacy	*Healthy lifestyles* Measures include tobacco use, physical activity, food choices and alcohol and illicit drug use	*Social outcomes* Measures include quality of life, functional independence, social capital and equity
Social mobilisation Examples include community development, group facilitation and technical advice	*Social action and influence* Measures include community participation, community empowerment, social norms and public opinion	*Effective preventive health service* Measures include access to and provision of relevant and preventive services	
Advocacy Examples include lobbying, political organisation and activism, and overcoming bureaucratic inertia	*Healthy public policy and organisational practice* Measures include policy statements, legislation, regulation and resource allocation organisational practices	*Healthy environments* Measures include safe physical environment, supportive economic and social conditions, good food supply and restricted access to tobacco/alcohol	*Health outcomes* Measures include reduced morbidity, reduced disability and avoidable mortality

Figure 1.2 Health promotion actions and outcomes

and are represented as *healthy lifestyles* in the model. The physical environment can limit access to facilities, or represent a direct hazard to the physical safety of people; and economic and social conditions can limit people's participation in society. These determinants are represented as *healthy environments*. These environments can both have an impact directly on health and social outcomes, and indirectly influence healthy lifestyles by making individual behaviours more or less attractive (e.g. by limiting or enhancing access to facilities for physical activity). Access to and appropriate use of health services are acknowledged as an important determinant of health status and are represented as *effective preventive health services*.

Health promotion outcomes refer to modifiable personal, social and environmental factors, which are a means to changing the determinants of health (intermediate health outcomes). They also represent the more immediate results of planned health promotion activities. Thus the cognitive and social skills that determine the motivation and ability of individuals to gain access to, understand and use information in ways that promote and maintain good health are summarised as *health literacy* in the figure. Examples of health promotion outcomes would include improved health knowledge and motivation concerning healthy lifestyles, and knowledge of where to go and what to do to gain access to health and other support services. *Social action and influence* includes organised efforts to promote or enhance the actions and control of social groups over the determinants of health. This includes mobilisation of human and material resources in social action to overcome structural barriers to health, to enhance social support, and to reinforce social norms conducive to health. Examples of outcomes would range from improved social 'connectedness' and social support, through to improved community competency and community empowerment.

Healthy environments are largely determined by *healthy public policy and organisational practices*. Policy-determined legislation, funding, regulations and incentives significantly influence organisational practice. Thus examples of outcomes here would be changes to health and social policies directed towards improving access to services, social benefits and appropriate housing, and changes to organisational practices intended to create environments that are supportive to health.

Figure 1.2 also indicates three *health promotion actions*—what to do, as distinct from what outcomes are achieved. **Health education** consists primarily of the creation of opportunities for learning which are intended to improve personal health literacy, and thereby the capacity of individuals and communities to act to improve and protect their health. *Social mobilisation* is action taken in partnership with individuals or social groups to mobilise social and material resources for health. *Advocacy* is action taken on behalf of individuals and/or communities to overcome structural barriers to the achievement of health.

Figure 1.2 can be used not only to illustrate the linkages between the different levels of outcomes, but also *within* levels. For example, among the intermediate outcomes, action to create healthy environments may both be a direct determinant of social and health outcomes (e.g. by producing a safe working and living environment, or improving equity in access to resources) and separately influence healthy lifestyles (e.g. by improving access to healthy food, or restricting access to tobacco products).

Implicit in the figure is the notion that change in the different levels of outcome will occur according to different timescales, depending on the nature of the intervention and the type of social or health problem being addressed—an issue referred to later in this chapter.

There is a dynamic relationship between these different outcomes and the three health promotion actions, rather than the static, linear relationship that might be indicated by the model in Figure 1.2. Health promotion action can be directed to achieve different health promotion outcomes by shifting the focus or emphasis to an intervention.

Scientists have attempted to describe the interrelationships between these different health promotion actions in Figure 1.2 through theories and models such as social cognitive theory and the transtheoretical model (stages of change). Increasingly, broader theories, using a social ecology framework, allow the inclusion of environmental and social influences to be considered in intervention design.

These theories help explain and predict how different health promotion actions can be directed to achieve different program objectives by shifting the focus or balance of actions. For example, efforts to promote healthy nutrition can be directed at the consumer as an individual using traditional educational communication, or at food manufacturers and retailers to improve the supply and promotion of nutritious food, or at catering outlets (canteens, restaurants) to influence food preparation and supply. Further information on the theories and models that guide contemporary health promotion practice can be found in *Theory in a Nutshell: A Practical Guide to Health Promotion Theories.*

The interdependence of these actions makes it difficult to assess the individual contribution of any one of the actions, and poses real problems in the development of evaluation methods and the analysis of results. These challenges in evaluation design are considered more fully in Chapter 4.

Deciding on what represents the best starting point, and how to combine the different interventions, will be guided by established health promotion theory, evidence from past programs, and knowledge of the local context into which the program will be implemented.

The development of program strategies incorporating the right combination of actions in the right sequence completes the planning stage of the program, and should link clearly and logically to the program objectives identified in the first stage of planning. This is known as a 'logic model', which is a way of describing the changes that the program is intended to bring about, defining what will happen during a program, in what order, and with what anticipated effects. The development of a logic model is considered further in Chapter 3.

Some modification of the objectives may be required at this stage, together with refinements to the measures used to evaluate short-term program impact. Examples of some of these measures are provided in Figure 1.2. Measurement of impact and outcome is addressed in greater detail in Chapter 5.

A clear definition of the planned optimal structure and sequencing of the intervention is essential to the second step of the evaluation process. It provides a point of reference for evaluating the process of implementation that has led to progress (or lack of progress) in achieving program goals and objectives. This is described in greater detail in Chapter 3, and is an essential and compulsory element of any program evaluation. This process provides key information of great use to practitioners in refining and reproducing interventions in the future.

Resource mobilisation: creating the right conditions

This stage is not only concerned with obtaining the resources (such as money, staff and materials) required for the successful implementation of a program, but it also refers to the need to build capacity in a community or organisation so that a program can be introduced and sustained, and to generate and maintain the community and political support necessary for successful implementation. It may also involve different forms of **formative evaluation**, testing and piloting of interventions that are to be used as a part of the program. Formative evaluation is described in greater detail in Chapter 3.

This stage is concerned with creating the optimal conditions for a successful intervention. A *resource assessment* can include:

• assessment of financial needs;
• determination of the availability of human resources; and
• analysis of how to generate such resources.

In circumstances where the resource assessment or formative evaluation of methods and materials show that the available resources or community response do not match that which is needed, it will be necessary to reformulate the program objectives to better fit available resources, and/or clarify the types of action needed to secure the community and political support that will generate the resources and opportunities for action that are required.

> Failure to give sufficient attention to the resource mobilisation phase in the development of a program, including the pretesting of methods and materials, is a common reason for program failure.

This is especially the case when program delivery may involve working through other sectors, such as schools, worksites and different agencies of government.

As with the planning stage, good record keeping at this stage will provide important information for evaluation of the process of implementation that leads to the achievement of program goals and objectives. Further information on process evaluation is described in Chapter 3.

Implementation

The implementation of a program (stage 4 of Figure 1.1) may involve one or multiple strategies or components to achieve the program objectives and goals emerging from initial analysis of the problem and its determinants. Traditionally, health promotion interventions have relied heavily on individual change approaches and public education or communication as primary methods for improving knowledge and changing attitudes and behaviours.

Increasingly, health promotion programs involve other forms of intervention designed to influence the social, environmental and economic factors that determine health. This requires working with communities in different ways to mobilise social action, as well as advocacy for political and organisational change. Combining the different interventions to achieve desired health promotion outcomes is one of the greatest challenges for practitioners. For example, an individual program to reduce teenage smoking might consist of a combination of different health promotion actions, each with different expected outcomes:

- *education* of young people concerning the negative consequences of smoking, with knowledge changes as the expected outcome;
- **social mobilisation** of parents and other social role models to make smoking less socially attractive/acceptable to young people, with attitudinal changes in teenagers as the expected outcome; and
- **advocacy** for legislative action to reduce access to tobacco and exposure to tobacco advertising, with policy changes as the expected outcome.

Figure 1.2 describes these different health promotion actions, and the subsequent measures that can be used to assess their impact and outcomes. At this stage, the primary aim is to ensure that a program is implemented as closely as possible to the original plan. Evaluating the process of implementation is the key evaluation task at this stage. Further information on **process evaluation** is described in Chapter 3.

Evaluation

Although **evaluation** is shown as the final phases of the cycle in Figure 1.1 (stages 5, 6 and 7), it will be clear that different types of research and evaluation form an integral part of the whole cycle.

Health promotion interventions can be expected to have different types of impact and different effects over time. Consequently, different evaluation methods are used to measure impact and outcome at different stages in the life of a program.

Impact evaluation measures the achievement of short-term program objectives defined during the planning stage of the program. These first groups of impact measures are often termed **health promotion outcomes**, and examples of the different types of health promotion outcome are provided in Figure 1.2. As noted above, these health promotion outcomes are intended to lead to subsequent change in *intermediate health outcomes*, such as behaviours and environments, in ways that will ultimately improve health and social outcomes in the model.

Consequently, intermediate outcome assessment is the next level of program evaluation, involving the measurement of the impacts of programs on individual behaviour or the social, economic and environmental conditions that determine health. Again, Figure 1.2 provides examples of these intermediate outcomes.

Health outcome assessment is the final phase in evaluation and involves the measurement of long-term or endpoint outcomes. As indicated in Figure 1.2, these are usually changes in health status, quality of life or equity in health status. These **health outcomes** are based on evidence or theory-based predictions of the relationship between changes in the determinants of health and the final health outcomes.

Figure 1.3 complements Figure 1.2 by providing a model to illustrate how a comprehensive set of health promotion interventions might produce different outcomes over a period of time.

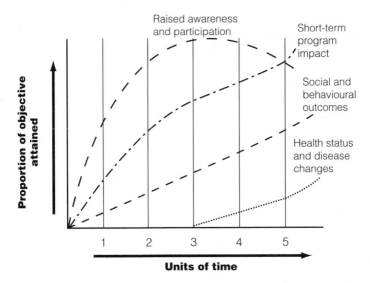

Figure 1.3 Theoretical distribution over time of outcomes from health promotion interventions

This model was originally developed to illustrate likely progress over a five-year period in a comprehensive, community-based heart disease prevention program. Thus, the 'units of time' are years, and the model shows how, after one year, the program impact could be measured mainly in terms of increased community awareness and participation in intervention components. By year 3, good progress in achieving short-term program impacts (health promotion outcomes) should be measurable, alongside peak-level community awareness and participation. Early progress in achieving intermediate outcomes (such as reduced behavioural risks) should also be measurable. After five years, major progress in these intermediate outcomes should be observable, and early impact on disease outcomes may also be observed.

This type of model can be of great use in explaining to program funders and decision makers the different measures of impact and outcome that can be used to assess progress, and the time required to produce different outcomes. This can be invaluable in managing expectations and promoting fairness in accountability for success over time.

The model in Figure 1.3 can be adapted to fit different types of intervention and different intensity of intervention. For example, an intensive public education program to promote uptake of a new childhood vaccine may achieve very rapid progress in raising awareness, achieving behaviour change (a simple one-off action is required), and achieving health outcomes (reduced vaccine-preventable disease), all within a matter of months not years. Similarly, a successful smoking cessation program for pregnant women, or a falls prevention program in the elderly, could more rapidly show health outcomes in terms of improved infant birth weight, or reduced injuries in older people. In these examples, the 'units of time' may be months, not years.

Summary

The planning and evaluation cycle (Figure 1.1) illustrates the different stages and their relationships in the development of a plan of action, implementation of a plan and assessment of desired health outcomes. These processes in turn lead to a redefinition of the priority problems and solutions, and hence the concept of a cycle of planning and evaluation. Because there are several stages, and often a long time delay between implementation and outcome, it is generally difficult to prove a causal relationship between actions and these long-term outcomes. It is essential that relevant and valid measurements are used to chart progress at each stage in the process. Adopting a systematic approach to planning helps to unravel some of these complexities and makes the identification of relevant measures of progress more straightforward.

The planning cycle summarised in Figure 1.1 will not address all the issues likely to arise in the planning and evaluation of a health promotion program. Real-life decision making never follows such a smooth path. This cycle, and the model outcomes described in Figure 1.2, is intended as a guide, to be adapted to prevailing circumstances rather than adopted wholesale without critical examination of its usefulness. In reality, few programs have the resources to apply this model in the systematic way described.

It is therefore important to identify what is possible, make explicit the program's likely impact and outcomes, and constraints, and indicate alternative ways to strengthen the intervention. The description of outcomes over time, illustrated in Figure 1.3, can be of help in communication with key stakeholders as to reasonable expectations of achievement over time, and form a basis for periodic program review and accountability.

> In order to plan and perform a high-quality evaluation, it is important to know the limitations of what can be achieved by the program under different circumstances.

The explicit communication of these limitations also helps to set realistic public and political expectations, thereby increasing the program's chances of success.

Further reading

Nutbeam, D. (1998), 'Evaluating Health Promotion: Progress, Problems and Solutions', *Health Promotion International*, 13(1), pp. 27–44.

Nutbeam, D., Harris, E. (2004), *Theory in a Nutshell: A Practical Guide to Health Promotion Theories*, McGraw-Hill, Sydney.

Rossi, P.H., Lipsey, M.H., Freeman, H.E. (1999), *Evaluation: A Systematic Approach*, 6th edn, Chapters 1–4, Sage Publications, Thousand Oaks, California.

Chapter 2
Key stages, methods and types of evaluation

This chapter provides an overview of the different research methods that support the planning process described in Chapter 1. It summarises the different stages of evaluation, and introduces different approaches that are described in greater detail in subsequent chapters.

Evaluation methods and types

Health promotion programs range in scope, scale, target population and settings. Four hypothetical examples of health promotion programs are described below. These illustrate the differences in scope among programs, and differences in the evaluation tasks required:

1. a small program encouraging people attending a diabetes clinic to take control of their condition and build skills that enable improved self-management, a feeling of greater control over the disease and its effects, and improved and healthier lifestyles;
2. a program encouraging Pap smear attendance (a behaviour to reduce cervical cancer risk) among a group of women from a particular cultural background living in one geographical area;
3. a program to introduce healthy menu choices and restrict smoking in restaurants and in worksites across a defined geographic region; and
4. a multiple-agency partnership, including departments of health, urban planning and transport, to use new urban designs for housing and recreational facilities to create a health-promoting physical and social environment.

The evaluation methods and the measures of outcome required for these programs will be quite different. Complicating matters further, in many health promotion programs there is more than one form of intervention and more than one evaluation method. Customised approaches need to be used to plan, implement and evaluate each program. For example, program 1 is set in a health facility, and has a small number of attending individuals to assess. A key evaluation challenge here is one of measurement—assessing if relevant measures (e.g. empowerment, self-efficacy) change in those who attend. The outcome to be measured is an improvement in measures of self-management of diabetes.

Program 2 is set in a multicultural community context, and will involve assessing the process of engagement with community stakeholders in the cultural group concerned. The evaluation will need to test how well health promotion workers engage with the community, and how well they develop and deliver a relevant Pap smear program to this community. The outcome to be measured is a sustained increase in uptake of Pap smears in a targeted group.

Program 3 involves engagement with many worksites/restaurants, defining program goals and objectives, and assessing how well an optimal program, given available resources, can be delivered to the participating organisations and their workforce. The outcome to be measured will be increased availability of healthy food choices in canteens, vending machines and restaurants.

Evaluating the effective functioning of partnerships is important when health promotion engages with other sectors, as shown in program 4. Assessing the common needs across agencies, and defining program elements in common, is a critical first step, followed by assessing how well the agencies work together towards a common task (in this case, the multiyear challenge of building health-promoting environments). The outcomes to be measured are multiple, and include changes to policy, changes to the built environment, and assessment of the impact of these changes on behaviours such as participation in physical activity.

The four programs will differ in the budgets available, the length of time available for evaluation, and the evaluation designs and research methods used.

Balancing scientific design with practical need

The introduction to this book indicated that the concepts of relevance, effectiveness and impact will vary among research scientists, practitioners, policy makers and members of communities that may be the subject of interventions. Health promotion research scientists will value optimal and tightly controlled research designs that are focused upon increasing academic knowledge and the scientific publication of results. These may have the best possible research designs, and provide evidence that may result from particular types of people participating in a program; typically volunteers in such settings have higher levels of education and health literacy, and are more likely to already be considering or motivated towards making the changes necessary in their lives or lifestyles recommended by the program. This may provide good quality evidence of program effects, but may not be 'generalisable' to the wider community; the same effects may not be achieved if the program were conducted in a poor neighbourhood, with diverse cultural groups or with the infirm elderly.

By contrast, evaluation that is usually under the direct control of stakeholders and practitioners has more flexibility in its approach, and uses opportunistic research methods to assess the program. This kind of evaluation is part of program planning. It first describes the program and its activities, and asks whether the program is useful and relevant for those who participate in it. This is typical for health promotion practitioners, for program managers and for members of the community.

Table 2.1 summarises key differences in perspectives by considering issues of control, research methods and desired outcomes. What will become apparent through an examination of the elements in Table 2.1 is that …

> … both science and practice are codependent, and are best served by a 'middle way'—an integrated approach—involving an evaluation partnership that meets both researcher and practitioner needs.

This approach seeks to understand not only the usefulness and relevance, but also the scientific value, of a program, and supports collaboration between researcher and practitioner towards this end.

Such partnerships, between funding agencies and researchers and practitioners, and between practitioners and the community/ stakeholders or participants, improve the quality of evaluation of health promotion programs. Health promotion science and practice can only advance if we know how and why programs work, whether

Table 2.1 The differences and similarities between practitioner and scientific perspectives of health promotion programs

Function	Practitioner perspective (informs program implementation)	Scientific perspective (provides scientific evidence)
Control of program, resources	Controlled by managers and/or stakeholders; evaluation carried out for accountability to funding agencies	Often externally funded by peer review scientific grant; designed and controlled by academic investigators with the purpose of furthering knowledge/scientific publication
Purpose of evaluation	Used to implement and improve programs, not to 'prove' that programs work; provides evidence on the need for more or different allocation of resources	Aims to generate scientific evidence for program effects
Research methods	Quantitative and qualitative methods; mix of research methods; triangulate results Apply pragmatic mix of evaluation methods based on needs/available funding May use mixed methods for assessing effectiveness of program; conclusions may include qualitative judgments of community/stakeholders	Usually quantitative methods; advanced statistical and methodological techniques; emphasis on statistical significance; conclusions flow logically from results Attention to methodological issues such as selection bias (who participates), measurement reliability and validity
Level of evaluation	Strong emphasis on formative evaluation, especially community consultation/needs assessments Emphasis on process evaluation—monitoring how well the program activities are implemented and delivered; may continuously change and improve program in response to process evaluation findings	Strong emphasis on impact and outcome evaluation and 'providing proof' or evidence of program effects Attention to the adherence to the research protocol ('fidelity' of the program implementation)
Research design	Flexible and pragmatic program design to fit the context and target groups addressed by the program	Tightly controlled research design, with greater measurable focus; may have single outcomes and shorter timeframes
Single focus versus comprehensive approach	Often multicomponent programs, with partnerships and interagency collaboration usual Duration: several years and interventions at multiple levels	May be single component or single focus for intervention in a specific group; often theory-based or testing a specific theoretical approach
Uses of results	Program failure leads to program improvement and modification; program failure may disappoint decision makers or the community such that funding or support are withdrawn Successful programs lead to efforts at dissemination more widely—to get the program used and adopted in other communities or settings	Contributes to scientific pool of evidence around the effectiveness of that type of intervention Successful programs need replication to examine if similar effects are produced in different settings or populations Programs that show repeated success amenable to: (a) meta-analysis to summarise results; and (b) dissemination trials

they are meeting the needs of communities and stakeholders, and whether they pass scientific scrutiny and critical judgment.

Stages of evaluation

Figure 2.1 provides the central framework for this book. It shows the different research and evaluation questions that are addressed stage by stage in the planning, evaluation and dissemination of a comprehensive set of health promotion interventions.

The first stages relate to the development and testing of an intervention, and later stages are concerned with the dissemination and adoption of effective or proven individual programs. Stages 1 and 2 indicate the importance of a range of different forms of descriptive research in the development of an intervention plan, as well as *formative evaluation* of the development of program components.

Stage 3—innovation testing—represents the evaluation of the effectiveness of an individual program. This includes *process evaluation* and assessment of the impact and outcome of the individual program (**outcome evaluation**). On the basis of evidence produced at this stage, decisions can be made on whether its use and adoption should become more widespread.

During stage 4 the intervention is replicated and tested in other settings to assess, for example, whether or not it works as well in other populations, or other places. Gradually, the emphasis on assessing the effectiveness of individual program evaluation elements is replaced by a focus on the process of implementation and the extent to which successful implementation can be reproduced and systematised so as to achieve the same outcomes.

By stage 5, the research focus is on the dissemination process, and on maximising the reach of the intervention—thereby maximising its potential public health benefit. This requires a focus on understanding the processes of implementation in different settings, and a decreasing focus on assessing the magnitude of the impact on outcomes. Stage 6, when a program is widely adopted, is the phase of program sustainability and maintenance (or program monitoring). This phase highlights the importance of continued monitoring of quality processes, but distinguishes between this more routine process and the more formal research and evaluation methods that are required in the preceding stages.

What will become apparent by considering the model is that different but connected research methods contribute to health

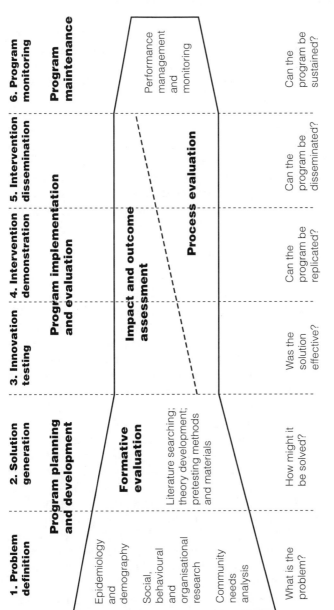

Figure 2.1 Building evidence for public health programs: stages of research and evaluation

promotion planning and evaluation. These range from using epidemiological studies (stage 1), through program planning and formative evaluation to test community responses (stage 2), to formal evaluation trials of programs (stage 3), and study of the process of program replication and dissemination (stages 4–6). Through such a process, individual ideas and theories can be developed, systematically tested and, if found to be effective, widely replicated to maximise public health benefit.

While not everyone can be an expert in all of the research methodologies implied in the stages of the evaluation model, it is important to have an understanding of the distinctive forms of research that support health promotion, and have the ability to critically analyse the quality and relevance of different types of research. Each stage is considered in turn, and is illustrated using published case studies from the literature on youth smoking prevention. These case studies are summarised in Table 2.2.

Stage 1: problem definition

The stage of problem definition concerns the use of different forms of descriptive data used in program planning. In particular, it requires familiarity with basic epidemiological research (such as causes of mortality and morbidity, identifiable risks to health, and the use of health-promotion-relevant prevalence data in populations). Specifically, **behavioural epidemiology**, which is the use of epidemiological methods to understand the origins and determinants of health-related behaviours, and *social epidemiology*, which explores evidence for socioeconomic and structural causes for preventable ill health, are important disciplines.

This research explores the issue, and investigates the causal basis and scope for a preventive or health promotion intervention. Relevant work includes conducting community needs assessments to identify community concerns and priorities, identifying access points to reach and work with key individuals and populations, and enabling more direct community participation in problem definition and solution generation. This information identifies the major health problems experienced within a defined population, the known causes of these problems, and the scope for change in those causal and contributory factors.

For example, the first case study in Table 2.2 (Currie et al., 2004) was based on a set of school-based surveys of adolescents across Europe. In 2001–02, over 35 countries or regions provided representative population data on youth risk and lifestyles. The

Table 2.2 Case studies of research that illustrate the stages in the model using youth smoking as an example

Stage of the model	Evaluation type	Principles underpinning case study	Case study
1. Problem definition	Formative	Youth population or school-based surveys, indicating the prevalence of smoking, age of onset, and subgroups at risk	Health Behaviour in School Children (2001–02 survey) in Currie et al. (2004) on smoking prevalence: based on representative samples of school-aged children (11, 13 and 15 years); asked a range of questions, including ever smoked, age of onset and current smoking status
2. Solution generation	Formative	Behavioural research to identify the correlates or determinant factors associated with youth smoking	Surveys of Californian Grade 8–9 students (Henriksen et al., 2004) showed that social influence factors (peer smoking and parental smoking) were related to onset of tobacco use; innovative questions also demonstrated a 50% increase in the likelihood of ever smoking for teenagers who regularly visited small shops that advertised and sold cigarettes
3. Innovation testing	Process/ impact	Examples of a controlled trial of smoking prevention and smoking reduction program among teenagers	A cluster randomised trial of smoking prevention in 30 high schools in Perth, Western Australia (Hamilton et al., 2005). The intervention school students, exposed to an innovative harm-minimisation curriculum (using a health-promoting schools model), showed lower recent and regular smoking rates at 12–18 months, compared to the usual school health curriculum in control schools
4. Intervention demonstration (replication)	Impact/ process	Replication of previously demonstrated effective smoking prevention interventions 'in real-world conditions with usual classroom teachers'	Earlier interventions in Minnesota (USA) and Norway had shown curriculum-based interventions to be effective for youth smoking prevention. This study (Nutbeam et al., 1993) was a controlled trial to replicate that approach in 'usual classroom conditions' in 39 schools in the UK. Schools were randomised to controls, family program, curriculum intervention, and both family and curriculum approaches. Rates of smoking adoption were similar across all four groups
5. Intervention dissemination	Process	Following the demonstration of an effective adolescent prevention program, efforts are made to disseminate it to a wider community	This paper (Hoelscher et al., 2001) takes an evidence-based school health promotion trial conducted in 96 schools, project CATCH (Child and Adolescent Trial for Cardiovascular Health), and assesses its implementation and uptake across three-quarters of all school boards in Texas. Subsequent communication with the authors indicated that in the five years since the 2001 study, CATCH was disseminated to over 1000 more schools in Texas, and 5000 schools across the USA, indicating that the process of dissemination was not static

study identified that one-quarter of 15-year-old youth were smokers, with the gender differences at age 11 (fewer girls than boys smoked) disappearing by age 15. There was substantial variation in smoking prevalence by country, region and social class. Parental and peer smoking rates were found to be consistently associated with smoking among the study population, but the importance of this link varied among groups. This data provides essential background information to inform program development by identifying key target populations (e.g. age, gender, place), and specific risks for smoking behaviour, such as the impact of national policies and programs, as well as parental and peer influence.

Stage 2: solution generation

This stage draws upon social and behavioural research to improve understanding of target populations, and the range of personal, social and environmental and organisational characteristics that may be modifiable to form the basis for intervention. This stage may also involve pilot testing intervention components. These methods of formative evaluation are described in Chapter 3.

At this stage, intervention theory development may also occur, to help to explain and predict change in individuals, social groups, organisations and the political process. Such theories and models are particularly useful in identifying plausible methods for achieving change in the personal, social and environmental characteristics referred to above, and the potential for general application in different settings and with different population groups. More information on intervention theory can be found in the companion book, *Theory in a Nutshell: A Practical Guide to Health Promotion Theories*. This information clarifies the potential content and methods for intervention, and further defines the different needs of populations.

For example, the second case study in Table 2.2 (Henriksen et al., 2004) shows cross-sectional survey data, which helps both with the clarification of the problem and with the generation of ideas to solve the problem—in this case, the development of an adolescent smoking prevention program. The study is from a survey of 2125 Grade 8 and 9 students in California to assess the influence of tobacco marketing on the likelihood of youth smoking. Students who regularly visited small shops where tobacco products were sold, or those who recalled cigarette advertising in magazines, were more likely to smoke, even when the known influences of parental smoking and peer smoking were taken into account. These findings suggest the need for environmental and policy interventions to restrict cigarette advertising or access by teenagers, in addition to the more usual youth tobacco control interventions directed at social norms and peer influence.

Taken together, research in stages 1 and 2 enables program planners to describe the cause, content, target population and method that form the basic building blocks for planning health promotion interventions. Such information will describe a problem, can identify determinants of that problem, identify individuals, groups, institutions and policies in a defined community that are most in need of attention, and, through this analysis, propose likely solutions. Potential solutions can be further refined through *formative evaluation* of program components and eventually defined in terms of the program objectives described in Chapter 1. As indicated, once such program objectives have been defined, evaluation of a program becomes more feasible. These program objectives are the immediate, short-term focus for impact and outcome evaluation.

Finding a successful and sustainable solution to a defined health problem requires the systematic development and testing of an intervention.

Stage 3: innovation testing

Ideally, in order to establish evidence of success, evaluation of a new program will go through different stages. Two different but related evaluation tasks can be identified, namely *process evaluation* (assessing the implementation) and *impact* or *outcome evaluation* (assessing its effects). These are discussed further below, and in Chapters 3 and 4. The relative importance of the two evaluation tasks will vary as an intervention goes through different stages of development. Figure 2.1 indicates the logical stages of evaluation beginning with a focused evaluation study to address the question of whether or not an intervention achieves its desired outcomes—did it work? The function of such studies is to assess the extent to which defined objectives can be achieved operating in the best possible conditions for success.

Such studies need to be developed in such a way as to meet tightly defined methodological standards. These are described in further detail in Chapter 4. This type of study tends to be of greatest interest to scientists who value these standards above other considerations. However, in order to meet such strict methodological standards, these optimally designed studies are often developed using a level of resources and methods that are not easily reproduced. For these reasons, such evaluation studies often do not provide the quality of information on the process of implementation that is required by practitioners to enable them to reproduce the intervention under less than optimal conditions. Hence, the need for further study, even if an intervention is shown to be successful in these optimal conditions.

The third case study in Table 2.2 (Hamilton et al., 2005) summarises an example of this type of experimental research. This study was a cluster randomised intervention targeting 13–14-year-old high-school students from 30 volunteer schools in Perth, Western Australia. Schools were randomly assigned to intervention or comparison schools so as to minimise the effects that self-selection might have on the intervention (self-selected schools are more likely to work hard to get a result). The intervention was innovative, and classroom based. It not only reinforced the behaviour of students who did not smoke, but also focused on reducing smoking and helping those adolescents who smoked occasionally to quit. It included empowerment strategies to enhance cigarette refusal and to reduce exposure to smoking environments. Comparison schools received the usual health information about tobacco.

Close attention was given to the measurement of smoking behaviour in the study, as well as other factors that influence smoking. Assessment of smoking and related factors was conducted before the intervention, and again one year after. A year after the intervention, regular smoking was lower in intervention than control school students (9.6% and 13.4%, respectively) and smoking in the previous 30 days was also significantly lower (20.4% and 25.3%, respectively). This innovative approach was more effective than smoking prevention programs using life skills or social influence approaches.

Stage 4: intervention demonstration (replication)

At the fourth stage of intervention demonstration (**replication**), a shift in the relative emphasis given to assessing outcomes and understanding process can be observed. If an intervention achieves the desired outcomes under ideal circumstances, the emphasis of the evaluation changes to consider more closely how to identify the conditions for success. Here the task is to replicate a program in circumstances that are closer to 'real-life' and that examines the type of issues that are important to health practitioners, such as the practicality of implementation of a program, and the extent to which a program can be adapted to meet variations in local need and circumstances. This is known as an **effectiveness** study, where an intervention is tested in 'real-world' conditions.

Such replication studies are often of great relevance to policy makers and program funders, as well as health promotion practitioners, as they indicate that desired outcomes may be achievable in circumstances closer to real life. Specifically, they take account of the contextual variables of health promotion practice, and indicate the essential conditions that need to be established for the program to be successfully implemented. Because of the balanced emphasis on both process and outcome, this type of study often produces more practical guidance (e.g. by indicating the importance of building community capacity and working across sectors), as well as clarifying the resources that need to be committed for success. This stage in the process offers the opportunity for assessment of costs and benefits more related to 'real-life' conditions.

Chapter 4 describes the range of issues that have to be considered in the design of this type of study, highlighting, for example, the tensions in maintaining the rigour in study design that is required to assess outcomes, while ensuring that the intervention is responsive to differences in local circumstances, and changes in the operating environment during the life of a program.

The fourth case study in Table 2.2 (Nutbeam et al., 1993) provides an example of this type of evaluation. Earlier work in Minnesota, USA, and in Norway had demonstrated that curriculum-based interventions, using contemporary teaching methods, were effective in smoking prevention among adolescents. This study was designed to replicate this type of intervention under usual classroom conditions with 'ordinary' classroom teachers in the UK. A cluster randomised controlled trial was carried out with 4538 students aged 11–12 years old from 39 schools to examine whether this intervention worked in real-world conditions. There were four groups: controls; a family smoking prevention program; the curriculum intervention; and, finally, both the family and curriculum interventions.

At the two-year follow up, rates of regular smoking were 11.3%, 14.4%, 12.0% and 10.1%, respectively, across the four groups, which were not significantly different from each other. All four groups showed similar increases in smoking-related knowledge and beliefs. The study demonstrated that replicating previously effective programs in real-world conditions may not be as effective as the original trials suggested. It provides an important reminder that …

> … we cannot assume that a study that works well in one set of conditions can be transferred to a different environment and assumed to have equal success.

Stage 5: intervention dissemination

The fifth stage—intervention dissemination—indicates a shift in emphasis still further. Here, attention is given to identifying the ways in which successful programs can be widely disseminated. Such studies include those directed at improving understanding of the ways in which communities can be supported to adopt and maintain innovations and build capacity, as well as studies of communities and organisations to determine how best to create the necessary conditions for success in different settings.

In this type of study the relative balance between outcome and process evaluation has moved further still. The primary focus is on the process of change, and research is directed towards assessing the success of dissemination strategies. This type of information is of great interest to policy makers and program funders, as well as practitioners, because it helps to define what needs to be done, by whom, to what standard, and at what cost. This type of research is least common in the health promotion research literature, partly as a natural consequence of decline in the number of interventions that reach this stage of development (i.e. of proven **efficacy**).

The fifth case study in Table 2.2 (Hoelscher et al., 2001) provides an example of this type of study. Project CATCH was a comprehensive school health promotion program developed and trialled in 96 schools across the USA (Luepker et al., 1996). It was shown to have good implementation, and produced effects on several health behaviours in upper-primary-school-age students. Immediately after the trial results, few schools adopted the program. This study reports on a partnership between CATCH investigators and the state health department in Texas to develop a dissemination strategy for the program.

Using *diffusion of innovation theory*, the researchers developed a partnership with a range of agencies, identified funding, and set about training teachers and engaging schools in adopting this evidence-based program. By the end of 2000, 728 primary schools had obtained the CATCH program, and teachers from 528 schools had been trained in its use. This study provides an example of the research and evaluation methods that can be applied to assess the dissemination of an evidence-based program across a whole region.

Stage 6: program monitoring

Beyond this stage, the basic evaluation tasks are directed towards supporting program management. These tasks include population-level monitoring of the outcome indicators of interest, and continuing performance monitoring of the quality of program delivery. Although this stage is not considered in detail in this book, the assessment of 'quality' in health promotion has been given considerable attention in the recent past, and a number of guides and manuals have been produced to assist with this task (see recommended reading). Methodologically, many of the tasks are essentially similar to process evaluation described in Chapter 3.

Similar to quality control in any system, this stage requires close attention to implementation according to established methods and standards of outcome. Good monitoring of professional practice, combined with systems for routine measurement of outcomes, risk factors and key determinants for health, are required at this stage.

Quantitative or qualitative methods in program evaluation

Both **quantitative methods** and **qualitative methods** can contribute to each of the research stages described above. In many circumstances, they are synergistic, and good quality evaluation has components of both.

> Qualitative methods are most often used in planning the program and defining target group needs, and quantitative methods in assessing program effects.

Quantitative methods underpin much of the published research in health promotion. These methods are derived from approaches developed in epidemiology, quantitative behavioural and social sciences, statistics and demography. They focus on numeric data amenable to statistical analyses, which allow a researcher the opportunity to test ideas regarding the comparison of some attribute between groups, the assessment of changes over time or the association between two or more measures. In this approach, statistical testing (based on the probability of finding a difference that you observe) informs the researcher. A statement that the improvement over time is 'significant' means that it is unlikely to be due to chance or random variation alone. More information is provided on statistical tests in Chapters 4 and 5.

Quantitative methods are used where numeric data is available, and statistical tests performed to provide evidence in a traditional scientific method. Quantitative research follows a set of logical steps, from defining a testable research question, through the steps of research design, data collection, data analysis and interpretation, to finally reaching a conclusion.

As an example, it might be shown in the evaluation of program 1 (referred to at the beginning of the chapter), on encouraging people attending a diabetes clinic to take control of their condition, that those attending the clinic make observable improvements in measures of dietary intake and measured body weight, compared to a group not attending the clinic, and these differences could be expressed statistically. Provided that the measures used are valid, this allows precise estimates of program effects to be made.

On the other hand, qualitative research methods have their historical roots in social sciences such as anthropology and political science. Methods include the use of focus groups (structured discussions with stakeholders or members of a target group), or directly learning from participating in or with target group members (ethnographic research or participant observation, sometimes called 'action research').

The processes of good qualitative research are the same as quantitative research, moving through logical steps from identifying a clear research question, data collection, data analysis and interpretation. The data (information generated from this process) needs to be analysed to give it structure, but are not directly amenable to statistical analysis. Thus, the original hypothesis (the idea that something may change following a health promotion intervention) is not proven or refuted through statistical analysis, but on the interpretation of the researcher, based on the rules for good conduct of the particular type of qualitative research undertaken.

These qualitative methods are useful where information needs to be elicited from individuals or groups that are not already well defined. For example, the women in program 2, referred to at the beginning of the chapter, may have culture-specific beliefs about preventive care such as Pap smears that will have an impact on the likelihood of their participating in any program. These beliefs may be related to the gender of their health provider or the perceived benefits of being screened, and the health promoter may be unaware of these issues. Qualitative methods will be more efficient at identifying these beliefs or concerns; this understanding would lead to the delivery of more effective programs, and the development of more relevant measures to assess their relevance and effects. The information obtained from qualitative methods can often feed into the development and refinement of concepts and measures that are used in the quantitative phase of the evaluation.

Another situation where qualitative research methods are useful may be in asking community members to describe the effects of a program, the barriers to participation or the strengths of program components. In such circumstances, statistical data is not required. In program 3 (referred to at the beginning of the chapter)—a program to introduce healthy menu choices and restrict smoking in restaurants and in worksites—stakeholder interviews with local restaurant owners could provide health promotion practitioners with useful information that enables evaluation of the effects and identification of barriers. For example, in a study of the effects of introducing a ban on smoking in restaurants (Lok et al., 1997), the researchers found that despite the restaurant owners understanding and accepting the health consequences of passive smoking in their restaurants, they were worried that imposing smoking bans would result in them losing too many customers. This information refocused the health promotion team to consider strategies to better enlist the support of restaurant managers. This provided a separate set of information on program effects to that obtained through quantitative methods.

Using data collection techniques that are less structured than those required for statistical analysis and allow a diversity of responses, qualitative methods provide a broader range of expected and unexpected information for program planning and assessment. This additional information contributes to a better understanding of the program, to explain why it worked and to define which program elements were perceived as successful.

Despite this, qualitative research is frequently undervalued and underused. Part of the reason for this stems from a value system that has evolved among public health researchers (especially those with substantial training in epidemiology and biostatistics), which gives quantitative research high status and tends to devalue qualitative research (frequently referred to as 'soft' research). As a consequence, such methods may either be inappropriately applied or, when properly applied, inappropriately assessed through academic peer review.

As indicated above, although the methods may be different, qualitative research can be planned and executed with scientific rigour similar to that of quantitative research.

> Identification of aims, selection and sampling of subjects, method of investigation and analysis of results can be as well defined and described in qualitative research as in quantitative research.

What becomes clear from this overview is that the best approach is to use both qualitative and quantitative methods. Neither is an 'easy method'. Since health promotion programs are often complex multicomponent interventions at many levels, it is appropriate to consider both, and to observe the program from a number of different perspectives. For example, if the qualitative semistructured interviews of women indicated that the Pap smear program (i.e. program 2, referred to at the beginning of the chapter) was culturally acceptable and easily accessible, this would be an indicator of success. If the quantitative data indicated increased understanding of the role of cervical cancer screening, and increased Pap smear attendance rates by women exposed to the program, then the quantitative data would corroborate the qualitative findings. Both taken together provide greater confidence that the observation of program 'success' is real.

This so-called **triangulation** of information from different sources can be a very powerful tool in health promotion evaluation and is considered further in Chapters 3 and 4.

Formative, process and outcome evaluation

Figure 2.1 also indicated the three key types of health promotion evaluation as formative, process and impact/outcome evaluation.

- *Formative evaluation* is directed towards answering questions of relevance to identified health problems, and the practicality of different intervention methods.

- *Process evaluation* is directed towards answering questions concerning the process of implementation, and recording the extent to which the program was implemented as planned.
- *Impact/outcome evaluation* is directed towards answering questions concerning whether the program successfully achieved its goals (such as changes in health behaviours) and objectives (such as improved knowledge and skills), as described in Chapter 1.

Formative and process evaluation form the central focus of Chapter 3, while research methods and designs for evaluating outcomes is the focus of Chapter 4. Chapter 5 examines the measurement of outcomes used in evaluation. Optimal (and well-funded) evaluations would include all three types of evaluation. Chapter 1 indicated that the process of evaluation is continuous, starting when the program is first conceptualised, and continuing until after the program has finished, and on further as it is replicated and disseminated into other settings.

In practice, time and attention are not necessarily divided equally among these evaluation types. Pilot programs need mostly formative work, while field studies in real-world settings tend to emphasise process evaluation. Health promotion interventions that are set up as research studies, or large-scale expensive interventions, warrant greater investment in impact/outcome evaluation as well, which may require technical design and statistical support from researchers.

The level of evaluation depends on the purposes of the program and also on its innovation. New programs that have never been tested should be assessed for their capacity to produce outcomes; existing programs that have been trialled elsewhere should be monitored to demonstrate that they are delivering programs of a consistent quality.

Summary

Evaluation of health promotion interventions is a complex enterprise. It is often done poorly, using methods and measures that are inappropriate for the stage of development of an intervention. Many of the problems faced by practitioners attempting to evaluate health promotion activity stem from unreasonable expectations of both the activity and the evaluation.

Not all programs need to be evaluated to the same level of intensity or using the same evaluation designs. The stages of evaluation in Figure 2.1 indicate how the evaluation question changes with the evolution of a program. The relative importance of formative, process and outcome evaluation will vary as the research question and the purpose of the evaluation change. The different stages of developing, testing, replicating and disseminating a successful intervention each require a different evaluation design, research methods and measures of success.

Both qualitative and quantitative research methods contribute to successful evaluations. In most cases, it will be important to use evaluation designs that combine different research methodologies. The generation and use of a diverse range of data and information sources will generally provide more illuminating, relevant and sensitive evidence of effects than a single 'definitive' study. Process evaluation not only provides valuable information on how a program is implemented, what activities occur under what conditions, by whom, and with what level of effort, but will also ensure that much more is learned and understood about success or failure in achieving defined outcomes.

Through this understanding, it is possible to identify the conditions that need to be created to achieve successful outcomes. Evaluations have to be tailored to suit the activity and circumstances of individual programs—no single method can be 'right' for all programs.

References

Currie, C., Roberts, C., Morgan, A., Smith, R., Settertobulte, W., Samdal, O. et al. (eds) (2004), 'Young People's Health in Context. Health Behaviour in School-Aged Children (HBSC) Study: International Report from the 2001–02 Survey', *Health Policy for Children and Adolescents*, No. 4, WHO Regional Office for Europe, Copenhagen.

Hamilton, G., Cross, D., Resnicow, K., Hall, M. (2005), 'A School Based Harm Minimization Smoking Intervention Trial—Outcome Results', *Addiction*, 100, pp. 689–700.

Henriksen, L., Feighery, E.C., Wang, Y., Fortmann, S.P. (2004), 'Association of Retail Tobacco Marketing With Adolescent Smoking', *American Journal of Public Health*, 94, pp. 2081–3.

Hoelscher, D.M., Kelder, S.H., Murray, N., Cribb, P.W., Conroy, J., Parcel, G.S. (2001), 'Dissemination and Adoption of the Child and Adolescent Trial for Cardiovascular Health (CATCH): A Case Study in Texas', *Journal of Public Health Management and Practice*, 7, pp. 90–100.

Lok, C., Bauman, A., Palin, M. (1997), 'Evaluation of the Chinese "Quit campaign" in NSW', *Health Promotion Journal of Australia*, 7, pp. 67–9.

Luepker, R.V., Perry, C.L., McKinlay, S.M., Nader, P.R., Parcel, G.S., Stone, E.J. et al. (1996), 'Outcomes of a Field Trial to Improve Children's Dietary Patterns and Physical Activity: The Child and Adolescent Trial for Cardiovascular Health, CATCH "Collaborative Group", *JAMA*, 275(10), pp. 768–76.

Nutbeam, D., Macaskill, P., Smith, C., Simpson, J.M., Catford, J. (1993), 'Evaluation of Two School Smoking Education Programmes Under Normal Classroom Conditions', *BMJ*, 306, pp. 102–7.

Further reading

Glasgow, R.E., Lichtenstein, E., Marcus, A.C. (2003), 'Why Don't We See More Translation of Health Promotion Research to Practice? Rethinking the Efficacy-to-Effectiveness Transition', *American Journal of Public Health*, 93, pp. 1261–7.

McDavid, J.C., Hawthorn, L.R.L. (2006), *Program Evaluation and Performance Measurement: An Introduction to Practice*, Sage Publications, Thousand Oaks, California.

Windsor, R.A. (ed.) (2004), *Evaluation of Health Promotion, Health Education and Disease Prevention Programs*, 3rd edn, McGraw-Hill, New York.

Chapter 3
Formative and process evaluation

Formative evaluation: testing methods and materials

Chapters 1 and 2 have shown that the evaluation cycle for a health promotion program starts with the generation of ideas to solve identified public health problems. These ideas may emerge from analysis of the problem or be obtained from previously published scientific literature, or from colleagues or other sources. This initial idea needs to be tested and explored to determine the elements of a program that might solve the identified problem. This first stage of evaluation is described as *formative evaluation*, which is a set of activities designed to develop and pretest program materials and methods. This is distinct from *process evaluation*, which is a set of activities directed towards assessing progress in program implementation.

Formative evaluation occurs as part of program planning, and before any elements of the program are implemented. This stage of program planning should occur in consultation with stakeholders and/or with members of the population who are the target for the program. Through this process of **participatory planning**, the key methods and materials that form an intervention are identified. The purpose of formative evaluation is to use a range of quantitative and qualitative methods to define the elements likely to be effective in the program.

Table 3.1 provides several case studies of health promotion interventions that have used formative evaluation to shape intervention methods and the development of support materials. These case studies illustrate the use of formative evaluation in both large-scale community trials, as well as the developmental work that underpins smaller health promotion programs. They also illustrate the range of possible research methods and settings for formative evaluation.

Table 3.1 Examples of formative evaluation in published health promotion papers

Author (year)	Context, program description	Way in which formative research was carried out	Influence of formative research findings
Jack et al. (2005)	Development of a mass media campaign to address the problem of binge drinking among Canadian youth	Six focus groups ($n = 66$) of Canadians aged 19–24 years; exposed to draft media messages and themes; asked about message dissemination strategies	Identified television programs suitable for dissemination; clarified terms for messages (e.g. 'binge drinking' not an appropriate term); identified campaign role models
Casebeer et al. (2003)	Design of tailored web-based educational materials for physicians about chlamydia	Followed optimal design principles for tailored web-based education; conducted needs assessment; pilot tested different modes of delivery and web formats	Tested registration numbers and engagement by physicians in pilot program; tested impact on knowledge in pilot group; identified best practice modes for physician education delivery
Caberra et al. (2002)	Designing a tuberculosis (TB) information and education booklet/resources for Latino Americans in USA	'Fotonovelas' style tested among low literacy Hispanic immigrants; needs assessment (TB patient survey); development of booklets with soap opera stories—tested with focus groups; review by TB professionals; field testing of revised resources with 13 patients	Health promotion resources need to be developed and field tested prior to dissemination, especially for culturally diverse groups
Manandhar et al. (2004)	Context is Nepal, poor maternal and infant health outcomes; program uses a 'community participation education model' to improve maternal and infant health; strong research design—randomised cluster trial	Participatory model (theory); program used facilitator training and participatory group sessions among women in intervention villages to define local needs and to develop ways of increasing skills among local women; developed programs in consultation with key village women (stakeholders)	Formative work resulted in similar (but locally relevant) village-level interventions; program resulted in better antenatal care and hygiene in intervention villages, and 30% reduction in neonatal mortality and 76% reduced risk of maternal mortality
Boyd and Windsor (2003)	Work towards the development of a food and nutrition program targeting disadvantaged pregnant mothers in Mississippi, USA	Community needs assessment defines problem as a community concern; this research identified the potential curriculum elements; the feasibility of using peer educators in the community; whether recruitment would be likely to attract target audience; piloting of 12 group-session curriculum; responses of target group women to pilot	Worked with stakeholders to define content areas of need; recruited five peer educators from community; pilot program trialled in small sample; focus groups post-program indicated loss of interest over time; confirmed by sequential drop-out of women through the 12 sessions; main result—that a shorter, less demanding, program was more likely to succeed (a six-session version was then developed)

For example, both the project to develop educational programs and resources for physicians, and the project to develop health education resources for Latino Americans, used extensive **consultation** with their respective target groups (Casebeer et al., 2003; Caberra et al., 2002). The purpose of the consultation was to gather information that would assist in the design of resources that target group members would find relevant, interesting, culturally acceptable and engaging.

Sometimes this formative evaluation will expose differences in the interpretation of priorities for action between 'experts' or researchers compared to the target group.

> Understanding the needs of the target audience, and using formative research to develop appropriate and accepted intervention methods and materials, is an essential first step in designing an effective intervention.

This type of formative evaluation will help to improve understanding of the way in which communities or groups experience and perceive health issues, especially concepts of risk and prevention. For example, the study by Jack et al. (2005) in Table 3.1 was intended to improve understanding of the issues surrounding binge drinking among Canadian adolescents. Previous interventions to reduce binge drinking have generally been ineffective, so better understanding of the beliefs and concerns of youth are required before new programs are developed. In this study, focused discussions were conducted with groups of Canadians aged 19–24 years to explore their perceptions of binge drinking and their views of strategies to address the problem. This information was used to develop mass media messages for a campaign, aimed at raising awareness among all Canadian youth.

In this example, the formative research enabled the development of clear communication goals, with simple messages targeting the beliefs and behaviours of these adolescents. Formative evaluation tested which messages to use, and whether they were understood, clear, and perceived as appropriate for their intended audience—and which channel of media message delivery would be most effective in reaching the target audience. This example provides an important reminder that there are many design principles for resource development that can be considered at this stage. These include the readability of the material (so that the audience could understand the message), cultural acceptability, and layout and design features. This applies to print media, such as brochures, pamphlets and billboards, and to electronic media, including radio, television and web-based resource development.

The consultation with community stakeholders to jointly develop a program to improve maternal and child health described by Manandhar et al. (2004) provides an illustration of a more overt partnership between health education 'experts' and the target population. Qualitative research methods (focus group discussions) were used in this example with mothers in villages in Nepal to facilitate the development of locally relevant maternal and child health programs. Using the information gathered through **structured discussion**, each program was individualised to the local village community context and needs. Aspects of program delivery were discussed, so that consumers would be more likely to participate in the programs that were offered. The challenges to implementation were discussed, and the literacy and beliefs of local women explored.

Using this method, effective lay-led health promotion programs were delivered across villages in Nepal. This formative evaluation can be part of a much larger community evaluation design, as shown in this example in Nepal, where the community consultation and program development preceded the cluster randomised controlled trial design for evaluating outcomes of this program (Manandhar et al., 2004).

A similar formative evaluation approach was used in the development of peer-led food and nutrition education programs in Mississippi (Boyd & Windsor, 2003). Here the content of the program and piloting of draft materials with small groups of disadvantaged mothers enabled the development of a structured 'curriculum', and subsequent refinement, as additional program elements were added to meet target group needs.

In each of these cases, the authors drew on existing theories to guide the development of their programs, and adapted these theories to fit the circumstances in which the intervention was to be delivered. Formative evaluation can also be used to develop and test new theories. For further information on the range of theories commonly used in health promotion, refer to the companion publication, *Theory in a Nutshell: A Practical Guide to Health Promotion Theories*.

In considering program planning in Chapter 1, we recognised that, despite the best intentions, in many cases practitioners find themselves under pressure to deliver a program quickly and may neglect to consider the preparatory work required before the start of the program. These examples demonstrate how important formative evaluation can be to the development of a relevant and appropriate program.

Although it will not always be possible to conduct well-structured and rigorous formative evaluation, as those illustrated in the examples in Table 3.1, it is an essential first step in the evaluation process.

> Undertaking formative evaluation will significantly determine the likelihood of subsequent success and failure, as well as building a sound basis for subsequent process and outcome evaluation.

Logic models

Building on the health promotion planning and evaluation cycle (Figure 1.1) and the actions and outcomes model provided in Chapter 1 (Figure 1.2), many find it helpful to develop a **logic model** of how the program elements are thought to work at this formative stage in the development of an intervention. This is a conceptual 'roadmap' or illustration of how the program elements might work. It is also a visual map, and conceptually depicts program logic, from inputs and activities (program components) through to the outputs and outcomes for each component. For example, a logic model shows the steps in the program, and what each might achieve. It illustrates the hypothesised connections between program components, and describes how program goals and objectives might be achieved. It is a planning tool, often drawn up in partnership with stakeholders, to describe the expected program effects at each level.

A logic model should consider the program inputs (human, financial and material resources), the context of the program (those factors that will influence the implementation and impact of the intervention, including the physical environment, social norms, political and community support), and describes the activities that together make up the intervention (e.g. program events, groups, training and social marketing). In turn, these are linked to the levels of outcomes that these 'inputs' are expected to produce (described in Chapter 1, Figure 1.2).

The development of a logic model at this stage in the process enables the person who is planning an intervention to structure the various sources of information that have informed the development of the intervention, and then to consider in a logical sequence the likelihood of achieving the program goals and objectives through each step and strategy planned for the program. It represents an extension of the ideas illustrated in Figure 1.3 in Chapter 1 by providing a more structured description of how the impacts and outcomes from a health promotion intervention develop over time, and providing a useful tool to manage the expectations of the community and program stakeholders.

An example of a logic model for health promotion is shown in Table 3.2. This adapts a logic model to the framework for outcomes described in Chapters 1 and 2.

The logic model shown in Table 3.2 describes a hypothetical program with the goal of improving the quality of food sold in school canteens in a region or school district. The structure of this example uses health promotion approaches: education and communication, and advocacy for structural reorganisation and policy development. Ideally, each of these different health promotion approaches would have been tested through formative evaluation with the target populations.

The logic model then uses the feedback from the formative evaluation to refine and define the intervention activities and, on the basis of the feedback from formative research, predicts the likely impact and outcomes. In this case, the short-term impact/outcome measures include observable change in food choices among students, favourable views of the program among teachers, and environmental and policy changes to support better food choices for students.

> Fundamentally, a logic model describes how the intervention elements might cause the program goals and objectives to be achieved.

Developing a logic model can be seen as a conclusion to the formative phase of evaluation—in this case, testing the conceptual framework describing possible program effects. If any stages are seen

Table 3.2 Hypothetical logic model: applied to school canteen menu and food improvement program in primary schools

| Resources and inputs | State education department, health department, school parent and teacher groups | | | |
Activities	Education	Communication	Organisation development	Intersectoral/policy development
Inputs	Teacher time; parents, canteen managers and suppliers	Teachers, parent and teacher groups, marketing professionals, media chosen (e.g. billboards)	Planning meetings; formation of steering group; garnering resources	Within-school reorientation to health/nutrition as priority issue; reach out to parents; food suppliers
Activities	Curriculum development; pilot testing through focus groups of students	Development of media resources (formative evaluation testing with students)	Planning meetings held; planning/logic model developed	School council or students' council makes policy changes regarding healthy nutrition
Outputs	Best practice curriculum for 'healthy eating' written	Campaign slogan and posters for all school canteens	Coalition of agencies formed	Planning group working with canteen
Intermediate effects	Program implemented in schools and awareness of program by students	Posters in all canteens; teachers aware of and accept the program	Healthy choices approved for canteens	Steering group work towards policy for healthy choices in all schools
Short-term impact/outcomes	Attempts at behaviour change; healthy eating choices increased among students	Parents and teachers have more favourable views of the program; parents' advocacy for the program increases	Working groups influence local food environment in schools	Policies around healthy food choices adopted in schools
Health and social outcomes	Reduced obesity and cardiovascular risk among children	Increased sense of school community generalises to other issues	Sustained healthy food choices due to widespread policy adoption	Health department and education department work together around other issues

as unachievable or unrealistic, then adjustments to the model can occur prior to that set of activities being implemented.

Overall, any logic model is conceptual, and developed at the outset. Subsequent practical experience in implementing an intervention may result in further amendment of the model.

Process evaluation: assessing implementation

Process evaluation is a set of activities directed towards assessing progress in program implementation. Process evaluation describes and explains what happens once the program has actually started.

It follows that the range of activities that comprise process evaluation is broad. Process evaluation identifies whether target groups were exposed to and participated in the program and whether stakeholders and partners were engaged with it. It also encompasses assessment of the short-term impact of an intervention—the *health promotion outcomes* referred to in Figure 1.2. Achievement of these outcomes is part of the 'process' of achieving the goals and objectives of a program that are described in Chapter 1.

> The aims of process evaluation are to understand how the program worked, what happened in 'real life', and how people reacted to it.

These are intervening steps in the processes of change. Understanding these processes is the most fundamental aspect of any health promotion program evaluation. Put simply, it is futile to expect successful program outcomes if the program has not reached the target groups, involved the appropriate stakeholders or engaged with the community as intended. It is an integral part of an experimental intervention (stage 3, Figure 2.1, and Chapter 4) to assess whether the different program elements were delivered as intended. It is also an essential part of stage 4 studies of replication/reproducibility (Figure 2.1). Here the evidence for program effectiveness is acknowledged through earlier studies, and the process of assessing the **reach**, adoption and utilisation of the program is assessed.

Process evaluation is essential in gaining an understanding of the mechanisms of dissemination of programs to wider settings (stage 5, Figure 2.1), to identify whether the effective parts of the program (e.g. adherence to a curriculum or structured learning activity) are maintained when the program has diffused into multiple environments in the field. For example, an evidence-based health promotion program may be developed and trialled in one set of schools but, when it is implemented across a state or region to many schools, it will inevitably undergo some local adaptation. Recording these adaptations, and analysing their potential impact on the program's effectiveness, is at the core of the evaluation of the successful dissemination of the program. This is sometimes referred to as assessing *program fidelity*.

Disappointingly, process evaluation is often not conducted to a high standard. For understandable reasons (pressure to demonstrate results), the resources available for evaluation are often exclusively channelled into outcomes assessment. This means that often we may not know how well a program was implemented, and consequently be in a poor position to explain why it was successful or unsuccessful in achieving predetermined goals and objectives. This knowledge is vitally important for practitioners. If a program has been successful, good process evaluation will identify *how* it worked, providing explanatory information, and identifying the mechanisms through which successful programs might operate. Alternatively, if a program fails to meet predetermined goals and objectives, process evaluation can help to identify the potential causes of failure, and support subsequent modification to improve the likelihood of success.

Monitoring the process is of importance to managers as well. It provides rapid feedback on the quality and integrity of the implementation and identifies ways in which program delivery could be improved as implementation occurs. Process evaluation can identify whether resources were adequate, and whether the program could be repeated elsewhere. This enables managers to understand factors associated with program success or failure. It helps define whether an ineffective program should be repeated, with increased or different investment or targeting, or whether alternative programs should be considered.

Process evaluation can include a broad range of methods and measures, but the most common elements are:

- *Exposure*: assessing whether or not participants were aware of the health issue being addressed, and exposed to the program or messages being offered in response. Failure to achieve understanding and recognition at this most basic level will have a fundamental impact on subsequent participation.

- *Participation*: identifying how well individuals, relevant groups and organisations were recruited to the program. This could include recruitment of people with a defined health problem, community members, organisations such as schools or worksites, and the level of engagement of partner agencies and non-government organisations (NGOs). Rates of participation will clearly help explain the subsequent effects; low participation will predictably lead to poorer results, while high participation increases the likelihood of successful outcomes.

- *Delivery*: assessing whether or not the program was delivered using the methods and materials as designed (program fidelity). This might include assessment of the extent to which participants use the resources, attend classes or participate in community activities in the way that was intended. Systematic use of a logic model can provide a good reference point for the assessment of program delivery.

- *Context*: examining reasons why the program was implemented as it was. This will include examination of the context in which the program was implemented, taking into account such variables as weather, current influences on social opinion and changes to the physical environment, all of which may have an impact on participation and delivery. Variations from the original protocol and adaptation of the intervention to local conditions are common in health promotion programs. Systematic recording of methods and materials used in an intervention will help explain subsequent observed program impact and outcomes.

Table 3.3 provides some practical examples of steps in conducting process evaluation. The tasks in Table 3.3 reflect real-world examples of things that practitioners can do, and information that can be collected during an intervention as a part of process evaluation. Most of these activities involve collecting information, keeping logs of program activity, completing audits of program attendance and participation, and keeping structured records of engagement by stakeholders. There are no fixed rules regarding which program elements to monitor; however, any clearly articulated components of a program plan or logic model should be monitored.

Table 3.3 Practical tasks in carrying out process evaluation

Process evaluation tasks	Examples of what practitioners could actually do
Exposure to the intervention/ elements of the intervention	Assessing 'exposure' to the intervention by survey or by focused discussions or interviews with samples of the target group, or staff and stakeholders, to identify their level of awareness of the program, and whether they were exposed to it, recognised it or engaged with it
Participation (describing intervention participation rates)	Identify how many people were expected to participate; count the numbers actually attending; keep a record of the proportion who attended all sessions or events (how many attended only some sessions or none?); document if there were specific subpopulations who did not appear but were expected (e.g. people without cars, people from specific ethnic groups, frail elderly adults with reduced mobility); measure satisfaction or perceptions of the intervention quality with program participants, or measure engagement with the program among stakeholders; monitor and document staff time/engagement (e.g. did it take longer to run the intervention?)
Delivery of the intervention	Record and monitor the number of sessions delivered, the location and completeness of program delivery at different sites; record ways in which program delivery differed at different sites
Context of the intervention (this is about describing the different settings and contexts in which programs are delivered)	Keep a log of problems in the delivery of the intervention, difficulties experienced, barriers to implementation reported by staff; interview a sample of staff, stakeholders and participants regarding the environmental and social reasons, costs or other factors that might influence the implementation of the intervention; record ways in which the program was delivered differently in different settings (e.g. what happened when support materials were not available as required, or program materials were delivered to a target population in a way that was different from what was planned?)

The case studies in Table 3.4 illustrate these principles further. They are published health promotion programs where process evaluation has been an important and identified feature. The diversity of styles of and purposes of process evaluation are illustrated here. All process evaluations occur after the start of the program, and assess what happened during the period that the program was conducted.

Some studies, such as the community cardiovascular intervention in Holland, try to ascertain which parts of community engagement and intervention worked and why (Ronda et al., 2004). A similar post-hoc review assessed environmental changes to promote healthy nutrition in Maastricht in Holland; here researchers went back to the supermarket managers to ask them about the intervention period and their views on how the program was implemented and why some of the healthy food choices were and were not marketed as well as expected (Steenhuis et al., 2004). In this example, process research was actually carried out after the program implementation—the program team sought information from supermarket managers for the period during the program, and about marketing practices in their supermarkets.

These are important examples of the strong connection between process evaluation and the assessment of outcomes; good process evaluation of an intervention can help to explain observed outcomes, and help explain whether factors in the program implementation might have contributed to the observed effects.

Comprehensive and systematic process evaluation has been applied and well described in community-wide interventions, such as the large-scale cardiovascular prevention trials (Finnegan et al., 1989) and large-scale cluster randomised smoking prevention trials such as the COMMIT trial (Corbett et al., 1991). In the comprehensive community-wide Minnesota heart health program, Finnegan et al. (1989) reported on the development of systems of process indicators, which were collected across different years, different programs and in different communities and target groups. These sets of data described the participation and exposure to the program in detail, and helped explain when there were or were not changes in community-level cardiovascular risk factors (outcomes).

The COMMIT community-wide smoking prevention trial (Corbett et al., 1991) described some of the context factors that made implementation difficult. These barriers included the policy context and structural factors that impeded implementation, and lack of homogeneous implementation across sites or across professional groups. This detailed process evaluation clearly enabled practitioners to understand why aspects of this program did not work.

The paper by Baranowski and Stables (2000) also demonstrated the impact of the context in which the intervention was implemented. Careful process evaluation showed that the healthy eating initiative was implemented differently across schools and worksites. In worksites, this meant that it reached disadvantaged workers less well than white-collar workers. These factors help to identify the

Table 3.4 Examples of process evaluation used in published health promotion papers

Author (year)	Program description	Types of process evaluation used	Main findings and usefulness of process evaluation to this health promotion program
Ronda et al. (2004)	Dutch regional heart disease prevention project in Maastricht region	Steering committee (stakeholders) interviewed; number of planning meetings held; count of number of project activities held	Defined limitations to functioning of neighbourhood committees (understaffed); stakeholders rated community participation as 'not very good' and environmental strategies as 'not implemented'; these interviews helped understand the lack of outcome effects of the program; may take longer (years) to engage with communities
Finnegan et al. (1989)	Tracking the implementation of the community-wide Minnesota heart health program	Cataloguing of program activities related to community participation, skill-building activities and social support	Comprehensive system for documenting implementation established and used to monitor program goals and objectives; also used to communicate with community stakeholders about how different strategies were progressing (in real time) and make adjustments to improve the program's reach and relevance
Corbett et al. (1991)	Process evaluation—COMMIT trial (22 communities: 11 randomised to comprehensive adult smoking cessation and prevention activities; 11 control communities)	Multiple projects comprise process evaluation tracking (e.g. community analysis, media monitoring, community taskforce activities, community events, tobacco industry activity, audits of professional training)	Increase in tobacco industry activity in intervention communities noted; tensions and local politics in taskforces slowed down programs; trial protocol adherence monitored in intervention sites varied (quality control review)—assessed 'dose of intervention' received for each intervention of 11 communities); validation studies to confirm self-reports of implementation; quality control of physician and other professionals' training in antismoking advice; attendance rates at 'quit and win' and other community events; ongoing surveillance to detect problems and intervene in real time to adjust program; understanding of external influencing factors, secular trends, competing community agendas and priorities documented
Steenhuis et al. (2004)	Evaluation of environmental change nutrition strategies at worksites and marketing healthy food choices at supermarkets	Interviews with managers at supermarkets about the healthy nutrition marketing and labelling program	Most managers had a 'positive opinion,' but indicated that healthy choice posters were the wrong size, labelling was not compatible with supermarket systems, program materials were not always displayed, there was a lack of time by staff and a lack of space in supermarkets, and the program did not attract customers' attention enough—these factors explained program ineffectiveness

Table 3.4 Examples of process evaluation used in published health promotion papers (*cont.*)

Author (year)	Program description	Types of process evaluation used	Main findings and usefulness of process evaluation to this health promotion program
Baranowski and Stables (2000)	Process evaluation of five-a-day fruit and vegetable project in nine sites in USA	Monitored each project with respect to recruiting participants, keeping participants, context of interventions, resources used; degree of program implementation, program reach and barriers	Settings (contexts) identified—schools, worksites; participation rates often lower than expected; in-school curricula were well implemented; worksite programs reached blue-collar workers less well; programs using social support, social networks or church-based networks showed good population reach; more research needed to define the quality of implementation
Steckler et al. (2003)	Process evaluation of Pathways project, a controlled trial of comprehensive nutrition and physical activity programs to reduce obesity among American Indian schoolchildren in 41 primary schools	Five major areas of process evaluation conducted: classroom curriculum; physical activity (PE lessons); food service changes; family participation; and student awareness	Process evaluation indicated excellent implementation: 95% curriculum classes implemented, and teacher surveys indicated strong positive views of the health curriculum; around 80% of PE implemented, with PE teachers supportive; 80% of food service staff attended training; around 80–90% of healthy food choices available to fourth and fifth grade students; 50–65% of students attended a family event; intervention school students much more aware of health program than control school students. Despite good implementation, objective changes in obesity not seen in the impact/outcome evaluation (Caballero et al., 2003)
Forster et al. (1998)	Developed local policy to restrict tobacco sales and implement policy to merchants; a community mobilisation project	Teams of 8–15 people developed/implemented program; uptake of smoking 'sales to minors' policy documented	All of the seven intervention communities adopted some degree of the policy; all banned vending machines; three warned merchants; and four fined merchants who sold to minors. Outcomes showed positive program impact, with students reporting reduced 'availability of cigarettes' in intervention communities, and a smaller increase in daily smoking noted in intervention over control communities

relationship between context (settings) and likely outcomes, and provide clues where additional support and intervention is needed.

The Pathways project, a school-based, obesity prevention intervention among American Indians, failed to show the predicted outcomes in terms of reduced obesity prevalence between intervention and control school students (Caballero et al., 2003). The study had exhibited excellent process evaluation, which indicated that the multistrategy program elements were carried out fully in accordance with study protocols, and community and teacher engagement seemed high (Steckler et al., 2003).

In this process evaluation, participation was high, indigenous cultural context was considered in the delivery, high rates of program delivery were achieved, and exposure was high. The findings clearly indicate that the program was implemented well, according to the program plan, and illustrate the difficulty in achieving obesity prevention outcomes, even where an intervention is well designed and delivered.

Finally, the trial reported by Forster et al. (1998) shows that policy implementation precedes reductions in youth smoking. In this trial, the policy adoption that occurred during the program period is an example of a process measure. The degree of implementation of the policy varied, but, in the intervention groups, policy change was implemented to some degree in all seven communities. The research design and measurements in this study were strong, so it provides encouraging evidence indicating that policy change can be causally related to a health behavioural outcome, at the community level.

Methods for conducting process evaluation

Table 3.3 described many of the practical tasks that can be undertaken in process evaluation. These may utilise both quantitative and qualitative measures. Quantitative data might consist of surveys or other instruments. Data regarding usage of resources, attendance at events or community coalition empowerment might be collected. Other kinds of quantitative measures of potential *mediators* might be at the individual level, and include increased understanding of an issue by participants, increased confidence by program staff, or increased community-level engagement with the program. For example, by assessing the engagement and practice of measures of professionals responsible for the delivery of programs, such as teachers or nurses, it is possible to determine whether or not they have low confidence or negative beliefs about the program, or have other constraints on their time that might compromise program delivery. The form of this quantitative data might include survey information that is analysed statistically or, more simply, counts or audits of attendance, participation or access.

Sometimes satisfaction surveys are used as part of process evaluation, but often suffer from biases, with many people unwilling to divulge program problems and difficulties. Such surveys will often produce 'positive results', with attendees describing how they liked the program, and appreciated the efforts of those who delivered the program. Unless very carefully conducted, this type of survey does not provide quality information on the process of implementation. Methods for reducing this form of bias are considered in Chapters 4 and 5.

In order to identify strengths and weaknesses of programs, it can be very useful to use qualitative methods. Semistructured interviews or focus groups with participants, and ideally some non-participants, can identify problems with access, language or program complexity that were not previously recognised; this can inform health promotion practitioners of issues *during the program*, and corrective action can be taken.

Researchers often wish to quantify the amount of the program that was delivered as intended (program 'dose'), the reach of the program (proportion of the eligible target group that participates) and the extent to which the program was delivered as intended (the *fidelity* of program delivery). For example, if half of the target group only attended two out of four classes, and a fifth attended none, then 'dose' can be accurately described, and outcomes examined in relation to the amount of program exposure.

The reach of the program is important for understanding generalisability. Estimates of program reach are important from a population health perspective, especially to identify if any subgroups were less likely to attend. These are often disadvantaged or marginalised subgroups, and it is essential to quantify their participation, as additional services or different kinds of programs may be required to meet their needs.

Summary

Despite the best intentions, in many cases practitioners find themselves under pressure to deliver a program quickly and may neglect to consider both the preparatory work required before the start of the program, and the importance of structured process evaluation.

Although it will not always be possible to conduct comprehensive formative evaluation, such as those illustrated in the examples in Table 3.1, it is an essential first step in the evaluation process. Undertaking formative evaluations will significantly determine the likelihood of subsequent success and failure, as well as building a sound basis for subsequent process and outcome evaluation.

Using qualitative and quantitative research methods, formative evaluation is the first step for testing the underlying need for a program with the target population. Formative evaluation provides a program planner with vital information to assess the feasibility of implementation of an intervention by testing the likely community response to planned activities. In practical terms, formative evaluation will enable development of the best possible and most relevant methods and materials for the intervention.

Careful and systematic process evaluation provides the foundation on which effectiveness can be assessed, as well as providing valuable insight on the practicalities of implementation—what activities occur under what conditions, by whom, and with what level of effort. This knowledge is essential for subsequent replication and dissemination studies. Information from process evaluation is also invaluable in interpreting the impact of evaluation data and its likely causal link to the program. Good process evaluation will ensure that much more is learned and understood about success or failure in achieving defined outcomes. Through this understanding it is possible to identify the conditions that need to be created to achieve successful outcomes.

By definition, process evaluation should occur during the delivery of the program. Process evaluation will describe what happens during the program and whether the program was implemented as intended. It can also provide a structured account of the elements in a program, assess if there was variability in program delivery, and identify the reasons for that variability. Process evaluation will also assess the reach of the program to its target audience, their awareness of the program, and their perceptions of the usefulness and relevance of the program. Finally, process evaluation will describe the strengths and weaknesses of the program, and explain why and how they worked or did not work.

Process evaluation should be regarded as a compulsory part of any health promotion program evaluation. Reflections on the processes of implementation can occur during an intervention, such that corrections and adjustments might be made in order to improve the likelihood of achieving desired outcomes. In addition, process evaluation data is examined alongside outcome evaluation data at the end of the intervention.

References

Baranowski, T., Stables, G. (2000), 'Process Evaluations of the 5-a-Day Projects', *Health Education & Behavior*, 27(2), pp. 157–66.

Boyd, N., Windsor, R. (2003), 'A Formative Evaluation in Maternal and Child Health Practice: The Partners for Life Nutrition Education Program for Pregnant Women', *Maternal and Child Health Journal*, 7(2), pp. 137–43.

Caballero, B., Clay, T., Davis, S.M., Ethelbah, B., Rock, B.H., Lohman, T. et al. for the Pathways Study Research Group (2003), 'Pathways: A School-Based, Randomized Controlled Trial for the Prevention of Obesity in American Indian Schoolchildren', *American Journal of Clinical Nutrition*, 78, pp. 1030–8.

Caberra, D., Morisky, D. et al. (2002), 'Development of a Tuberculosis Education Booklet for Latino Immigrant Patients', *Patient Education and Counseling*, 46, pp. 117–24.

Casebeer, L.L., Strasser, S.M., Spettel, C.M., Wall, T.C., Weissmar, N., Ray, M.N. et al. (2003), 'Designing Tailored Web-Based Instruction to Improve Practicing Physicians' Preventive Practices', *Journal of Medical Internet Research*, 5(3): e20.

Corbett, K., Thompson, B., White, N., Taylor, M. (1991), 'Process Evaluation in the Community Intervention Trial for Smoking Cessation (COMMIT)', *International Quarterly for Community Health Education*, 11, pp. 291–309.

Finnegan, J.R. Jr, Murray, D.M., Kurth, C., McCarthy, P. (1989), 'Measuring and Tracking Education Program Implementation: The Minnesota Heart Health Program Experience', *Health Education Quarterly*, 16(1), pp. 77–90.

Forster, J.L., Murray, D.M., Wolfson, M., Blaine, T.M., Wagenaar, A., Hennrikus, D. (1998), 'The Effects of Community Policies to Reduce Youth Access to Tobacco', *American Journal of Public Health*, 88(8), pp. 1193–8.

Jack, S.M., Bouck, L.M., Benyon, C.E., Ciliska, D.K., Mitchell, M.J. (2005), 'Marketing a Hard-to-Swallow Message: Recommendations for the Design of Media Campaigns to Increase Awareness about the Risks of Binge Drinking', *Canadian Journal of Public Health*, 96(3), pp. 189–93.

Manandhar, D.S., Osrin, D., Shrestha, B.P., Mesko, N., Morrison, J., Tumbahangphe, K.M. et al. (2004), 'Effect of a Participatory Intervention with Women's Groups on Birth Outcomes in Nepal: Cluster-Randomised Controlled Trial', *The Lancet*, 364(9438), pp. 970–9.

Ronda, G.M., Van Assema, P.T., Candel, M.J.J.M., Ruland, E., Steenbakkers, M., Van Ree, J.W. et al. (2004), 'The Dutch Heart Health Community Intervention. "Hartslag Limburg": Design and Results of a Process Study', *Health Education Research*, 19(5), pp. 596–607.

Steckler, A., Ethelbah, B., Martin, C.J., Stewart, D., Pardillo, M., Gittelsohn, J. et al. (2003), 'Pathways Process Evaluation Results: A School-Based

Prevention Trial to Promote Healthful Diet and Physical Activity in American Indian Third, Fourth, and Fifth Grade Students', *Preventive Medicine*, 37, s80–s90.

Steenhuis, I.H.M., van Assema, P., Van Reubsaet, A., Kok, G. (2004), 'Process Evaluation of Two Environmental Nutrition Programmes and an Educational Nutrition Programme Conducted at Supermarkets and Worksite Cafeterias in the Netherlands', *Journal of Human Nutrition and Dietetics*, 17, pp. 107–15.

Further reading

CDC Evaluation working group, Center for Disease Control and Prevention: Logic Models, http://www.cdc.gov/eval/resources.htm#logic%20model (accessed March 2006), produced by CDC, Office of Strategy and Innovation Evaluation Team, CDC Atlanta, Georgia.

Grbich, C. (1999), *Qualitative Research in Health: An Introduction*, Allen and Unwin, Sydney.

Steckler, A., Linnan, L. (eds) (2002), *Process Evaluation for Public Health Interventions and Research*, Jossey-Bass/John Wiley and Sons, San Francisco.

Chapter 4
Evaluation methods for health promotion programs

Chapter 3 described the different formative and process research methods that are used to support the development of a health promotion intervention, and to assess whether or not it was implemented as intended. This chapter focuses on the evaluation designs and research methods that are used to test the effectiveness of a health promotion intervention. 'Effectiveness' in this case means the success of the health promotion intervention in producing the impact and outcomes that were predicted during the planning of the program—the extent to which the program achieved its goals and targets, as defined in Chapter 1.

This chapter is focused primarily on research methods and evaluation designs required for stage 3 in Figure 2.1 (i.e. innovation testing). It also considers the different evaluation designs that are required for replication studies (stage 4 in Figure 2.1), dissemination studies (stage 5) and for assessing the quality of institutionalised programs (stage 6).

Evaluation designs for health promotion interventions

The term **evaluation design** describes the set of procedures and tasks that need to be carried out in order to systematically examine the effects of a health promotion intervention. Evaluation design encompasses all the steps required to understand whether an intervention produced the results that were expected. The purpose of a good evaluation design is to enable us to be as confident as possible that the health promotion intervention *caused* any changes that were observed. To do this we need to ensure that:

- the program was implemented as intended and reached the target audience (process evaluation—see Chapter 3);
- the best *measurements* possible were used to assess the impact and outcomes from the intervention (the results)—see Chapter 5 for greater detail on measurement;
- there are no alternative explanations for the results; and
- we can identify the individuals or population groups or subgroups to whom these intervention effects do and do not apply.

For example, in evaluating an intervention to promote regular physical activity we need to be able to:

- ensure that the physical activity intervention was implemented as intended by the program planners, and reached the majority or all of the target audience;
- measure changes in physical activity among the target audience using a valid and reliable measure of physical activity;
- distinguish between change that occurred as a result of the intervention, and change that may have occurred within the target audience had no intervention occurred (bearing in mind that people change their pattern of physical activity for many reasons, and not only in response to organised interventions); and
- clarify if the intervention was more, or less, successful among different groups of people (e.g. by being more successful in influencing physical activity among women more than men, or among specific ethnic groups, or affecting younger people more than older people, and so on).

Put simply, the better the evaluation design and methods that we use in assessing impact and outcome, the more confident we can be that the observed effects of a program were caused by the intervention and did not occur by chance, or were not due to other factors or influences.

As indicated in Chapter 3, the first step for any program implementation should be process evaluation, to identify whether or not the program was implemented as planned. This may require information to be collected on program attendance, participation rates among the target audience and identification of the characteristics of those who participated and those who did not. This data is an essential first step for all program evaluations. It is unlikely that a program will be effective in achieving the intended impact and outcome if participation among the target audience was poor, and difficult to assess the effectiveness of a multisite intervention if it was delivered in highly variable ways at different locations.

Careful and systematic process evaluation provides the foundation on which effectiveness can be assessed, as well as providing valuable insight on the practicalities of implementation that will be essential for subsequent replication and dissemination studies. In this context, information from process evaluation is invaluable in interpreting the impact evaluation data and its likely causal link to the program; if not well implemented, then impact and outcome data are seldom positive.

A broad range of evaluation designs has been developed for use in health promotion. This range of design options allows researchers to shape the research methods used to develop the 'best possible' design to match the context of the program, its implementation, and the expectations of the different stakeholders. For example, a program to increase the use of smoke-free policies in the workplace may have a different 'best possible' design compared to a community-based program to prevent falls in a group of home-bound older people. Each presents different challenges in relation to the process of implementation, the measurement of outcomes, and the management of the research environment.

The most commonly used quantitative evaluation designs are illustrated in Figure 4.1.

Experimental designs

The most widely acknowledged scientific evidence comes from *experimental* designs, commonly referred to as **randomised controlled trials** (RCTs). This is illustrated in design 1, in Figure 4.1. In this case, the population receiving the intervention is not predetermined. Individuals or groups are randomly allocated to receive the program, or not to receive the program. Every individual or group has an equal chance of being offered the program, or not. This *random selection* of individuals who may, or may not, receive an intervention minimises the possibility that observed changes in the intervention population occurred as a result of 'chance' effects that have nothing to do with the intervention. It improves confidence that the changes were *caused* by the intervention.

Experimental designs

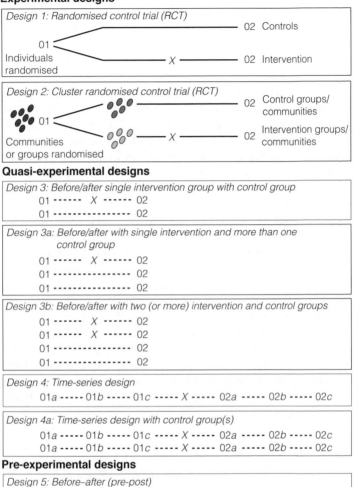

Quasi-experimental designs

Pre-experimental designs

Figure 4.1 Quantitative evaluation designs for individual programs (stage 3 of Figure 2.1)

Once the two groups of individuals have been allocated to receive, or not receive, a particular intervention, an assessment is made of the characteristics of the study population (such as age or gender) and the objects of the intervention (such as smoking behaviour or healthy eating patterns) to determine the status of the population *before* the intervention occurs. This is often done with a structured interview or questionnaire.

Sometimes objective measures are used, at both the individual and environmental level (see Chapter 5 for more on information measurement and the use of questionnaires). The same measurements are then performed on the same individuals *after* the intervention has been completed to assess change in the objects of the intervention. If the changes in the objects of the intervention (such as smoking prevalence or healthy diet) are greater in the intervention group than in the control group, then it is likely that these changes were caused by the health promotion intervention.

The importance of these findings will subsequently be assessed on the basis of the size of the change observed (i.e. the percentage difference), and the size and representativeness of the population that was studied in relation to the overall target audience for an intervention. *Sampling techniques* can be used to ensure that the population who is studied is representative of the whole target audience for an intervention, and *statistical tests* can be used to assess the importance (referred to as *significance*) of the observed changes between the intervention and non-intervention populations. These issues are discussed further below. In general, the larger the study population, the greater the chance of showing a statistically significant difference between the intervention and non-intervention populations.

In summary, the quality of the results from an optimal evaluation design are determined by:

- random allocation of the study population to intervention and control (comparison) groups to ensure that those exposed to the intervention are as similar as possible to those not exposed to the intervention;
- measurement of the characteristics of the study sample (intervention and control groups) before the intervention is implemented;
- use of a sufficient number of subjects in both the intervention and control groups (sample size) to detect expected effects;
- the implementation of the health promotion intervention (as planned) with the intervention group;

- measurement of the same groups using the same measures after the intervention is completed (ensuring that all subjects are included regardless of exposure to the intervention);
- analysis of the observed differences between the intervention and non-intervention groups using appropriate statistical techniques; and
- the representativeness of the study group of the population from which it was sampled.

The two examples in Box 4.1 show randomised trials of health promotion programs. The first is an 'individual level' trial and shows a randomised controlled trial of a health education intervention to reduce sexual risk behaviours among African American adolescent girls. The second shows a health promotion program at the community level, where the communities themselves are randomised to intervention or control.

Box 4.1 Examples of randomised control trials

Example 1: Individual-level randomised controlled trial: reducing sexual risk behaviours among African American adolescent girls

A randomised controlled trial (DiClemente et al., 2004) targeting sexually active African American adolescent girls aimed to reduce sexual risk behaviours. Participants were recruited through community health centres from client lists, and 522 were enrolled in the trial. Subjects were randomly allocated to intervention and 'normal care' groups. The intervention was 4 × 4-hour group education sessions, with condom skills development and a focus on healthy relationships.

Relevant behaviours and individual characteristics were assessed by questionnaire before and after the intervention. Compared to controls, girls in the intervention condition reported that they were twice as likely to always use condoms in the past month and past year, and reported improved measures of empowerment regarding relationships. The results suggest that targeted, gender and culturally specific health promotion programs can impact on sexual behaviour, which is also likely to lead to reduced sexually transmitted disease risk and reduced teenage pregnancy.

▶

Example 2: Cluster randomised trial: a trial of the effects of an intervention to change tobacco retailing policy

'Tobacco policy options for prevention' (TPOP) was a community-level randomised trial of changes in local policy to reduce youth smoking and restrict access to tobacco (Forster et al., 1999). This is an example where allocation to intervention and control would occur at the community level, as the policy intervention would be implemented at that level.

In this study, 14 Minnesota communities were randomised to policy-changing interventions (targeting youth and merchants selling tobacco) and control communities. Randomisation of communities resulted in baseline matching of youth from intervention and control communities on smoking prevalence and tobacco access. The program used a direct action community organising model; implementation varied, as communities each developed their own approach to policy to restrict tobacco sales to minors, but all intervention regions implemented a policy framework, and no controls did so (process evaluation).

Analysis was of individual students' perceptions and tobacco purchasing attempts (adjusting for community-level clustering). Results showed a reduced increase in smoking among intervention community youth, and purchase attempts were fewer than in control region youth. It is important to note environment regulation through policy-changing efforts in this study was assessed using optimal randomised trial designs, and produced population-level effects greater than those produced in usual school-level interventions.

An important type of randomised trial used in health promotion is the **cluster randomised control trial** (example 2 in Box 4.1 and design 2 in Figure 4.1). Here interventions are targeted to individuals within defined organisations or groupings, such as schools, worksites or primary care clinics. The *cluster* design is where randomisation occurs at the level of groups or communities, which are randomly allocated to intervention or control conditions. This is necessary and appropriate where individuals within a community share features in common (are clustered). For example, within the same school, students are likely to share common influences on their health behaviour or beliefs. These common influences on students' behaviours and beliefs make it appropriate to consider them as a group in a research study, but this has important implications for the statistical analysis of results. It is an efficient design to randomise at the level of the group or community, but requires additional technical skills when the data is ready for analysis.

It is important to make sure that randomised trials are ethical, and that nobody fails to receive the care or attention that they need. In these circumstances, 'usual care' or minimal interventions are provided. For example, in a clinic or primary care setting, it may be possible to randomly allocate groups of patients with diabetes to receive a comprehensive education and skills development program, and others to be allocated to a control group, which may receive only their 'usual clinic care'. In such circumstances it is important to follow ethical protocols, and ensure that your evaluation study has received approval from an appropriate university or health service ethics review board.

It is also important to keep the people in intervention and control groups separated from each other as much as is practically possible. If they communicate, and share the information or resources that form part of a health promotion intervention, this will increase the chances that this non-intervention (control) group will make the changes (e.g. to physical activity) that are the object of the intervention. Such **contamination** makes it much more difficult to detect the effects of a program. This is often very difficult in health promotion programs that are designed to reach whole communities—hence the use of cluster RCTs as an alternative.

Although the use of experimental designs is always preferable, this kind of evaluation design is most feasible when programs are well funded, and when it is possible to allocate people or groups randomly to receive or not receive an intervention. This type of design is most necessary when the need for compelling evidence is essential. This might include circumstances where a program is being tested for the very first time, or is expensive (and would be costly to reproduce widely), or may be controversial, or considered risky.

Quasi-experimental designs

Given the diversity of settings and complexity of interventions, it is often not possible to evaluate health promotion programs using

RCT designs. Alternative designs provide less rigorous evidence of program effectiveness, but may be the most feasible in many situations. 'Best practice' in health promotion evaluation will always require consideration of the 'optimal against the possible' in evaluation design. These non-RCT designs are classified as 'quasi-experimental' and 'pre-experimental'.

Quasi-experimental designs have clearly defined *control* or *comparison* populations—a population who do not receive an intervention, and against which intervention group effects could be compared (Figure 4.1, designs 3, 3a and 3b). In this case, the population receiving the intervention is predetermined and non-randomly assigned, so there is a risk that any observed changes may have been influenced by differences between the intervention and control groups or communities, and not caused by the intervention.

As is the case with RCTs, the quality of the results from quasi-experimental studies is dependent upon the size and representativeness of the study population, the use of valid measures before and after the intervention, the completion of the health promotion intervention as planned, and optimal analysis of the observed differences between the intervention and non-intervention populations. The analyses may need to take account of the differences between groups, and adjust for them where possible.

RCTs rely on continued participation by the same individuals throughout the program—the pretest and post-test is done on the same people. This is sometimes referred to as a **cohort** study. Quasi-experimental studies may also involve the same cohort in the pretest and post-test, but can also include a different, randomly selected, cross-section of people from the target population to obtain pretest and post-test information. This is referred to as a repeat **cross-sectional study**, and, while feasible in many health promotion program evaluations, it is not as methodologically strong as a cohort study for explaining how people changed.

Quasi-experimental designs are often the most practical for many health promotion interventions. This is especially the case where interventions are directed at whole populations or regions (the allocation of individuals to intervention and non-intervention groups is impossible).

Box 4.2 describes the use of a quasi-experimental design to assess a typical community-based health promotion program designed to increase physical activity.

Box 4.2 Quasi-experimental design: promoting physical activity in the community

In a study to assess the effects of a community-wide intervention to promote physical activity, Reger and colleagues (2002) conducted an intervention in Wheeling (a small city in West Virginia, USA) and used a demographically matched comparison community elsewhere in the state. The choice of intervention community is non-random; this community was enthusiastic to plan and develop a program; in this situation, a key element is choosing the control community(ies) so that they are as closely matched as possible to the intervention community. Matching should be on size, culture, socioeconomic status and age distribution at the least. In this case, for a media campaign, they needed to have different media markets, so the intervention materials would not be seen in the control community.

The intervention, 'Wheeling Walks', used a social marketing campaign, community capacity building, community partnerships and environmental changes to encourage middle-aged adults to start walking for their health. The comparison community did not share media channels with the intervention community. Process evaluation showed reasonably good implementation of the social marketing campaign in Wheeling, and evidence of community coalition building and partnership formation (Reger-Nash et al., 2006). Impact evaluation showed changes in awareness and understanding in Wheeling compared to the comparison community, and also increases in reported walking for health. The analyses adjusted for differences between communities before concluding the campaign had produced effects on the population.

'Wheeling Walks' was a quasi-experimental design, using one comparison community. Reger-Nash et al. then conducted replicate evaluations in three other studies, each with one control and one intervention community. This was carried out in pairs of rural communities, and used an extended intervention model (Reger-Nash et al., 2006). All of these studies used a quasi-experimental design, but fit into the replication stage of evaluation (see Figure 2.1, stage 4), and the evaluation attempted to work out the differences in effectiveness compared to Wheeling Walks. This included substantial process evaluation in each intervention, as well as impact assessment.

Another type of quasi-experimental evaluation design is a **time-series design**. In this evaluation design there are multiple preintervention measurements, followed by the health promotion intervention, and then multiple post-intervention measurements (Figure 4.1, design types 4 and 4a). Here trends in an object of interest (such as smoking prevalence, or consumption of fresh fruit and vegetables) can be observed, and the intervention effect is judged by changes to the trend line.

For example, Box 4.3 describes the results of an Australian mass media campaign to increase uptake of Pap smear tests (cervical cancer tests), reporting on changes observed over time in Pap smear rates following the campaign.

Box 4.3 Quasi-experimental time-series design: mass media campaign to increase uptake of Pap smear tests

Time-series designs are useful where repeat measures of the same phenomenon at the population level are occurring already (e.g. through routine health service data collections). The evaluation can be assessed against the background of this routine data collection, and if sudden changes follow the intervention against a background of constant rates, then they are more likely to be due to the intervention.

Shelley et al. (1991) described the results of an evaluation of a campaign to increase Pap smear rates in one state of Australia; a comparison was another state unexposed to the campaign. The intervention was a mass-media-led effort to encourage all women to attend for a Pap smear screening test for early detection of cervical cancer. Primary care services were also included in the intervention.

The design was quasi-experimental, with one intervention and one control region, but there was a time-series dimension—monthly Pap smear attendance rates were collected for several years prior to the campaign, and changes in these monthly 'averages' were assessed in the campaign state compared to control. The techniques to do this included assessing the rate of change over multiple measurements, and the use of statistical (regression) modelling to assess if the rate of change was different over time—here the intervention region showed a sudden increase in rate which was large (of public health importance and statistically significant),

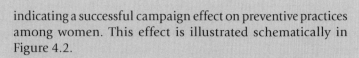

indicating a successful campaign effect on preventive practices among women. This effect is illustrated schematically in Figure 4.2.

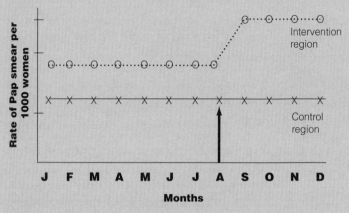

Figure 4.2 Time-series quasi-experimental design: effects of media campaign in August

The time-series design approach is strengthened by the addition of one or more comparison regions, which also have trend data (Figure 4.1, design type 4a). This is a quasi-experimental design, as the population receiving the intervention is predetermined and non-randomly assigned, so there is a risk that any observed changes may have been influenced by factors or events other than the intervention. As with each of these designs, the quality of the results is also dependent upon the size and selection of the study population, the use of valid measures and the completion of the health promotion intervention as planned. This type of quasi-experimental design is particularly useful where there are sources of data that are regularly collected by health authorities (such as Pap smear tests), or other government and non-government sources that can be accessed for use in this way.

Pre-experimental designs

The last group of designs have been described as *pre-experimental*. These provide the weakest evidence and should only be used when other possibilities have been explored.

A 'before–after' (**pre–post study**) one group design (type 5, in Figure 4.1) is a relatively weak design, as it can only provide observations about change in the objects of interest and, on its own, this type of evaluation design does not provide compelling evidence that a health promotion intervention *caused* the observed changes (as indicated previously, people change their behaviours for many reasons, and not only in response to organised interventions). Nonetheless, this simple evaluation design does give some estimate of change, and is often used in pilot studies to estimate the likely effect of an intervention.

Sometimes, a before–after design is the only design that is possible (e.g. if a large-scale mass media campaign is being implemented). Here, it may not be possible to have a comparison population or region, especially if the campaign is at the national level and targets the whole population.

In all evaluation designs that involve post-test measurement, the timing of the measurement of outcomes is critical. In Figure 1.3 (Chapter 1) we illustrated the distribution of outcomes following a health promotion intervention. Figure 1.3 illustrated how it may take many months, even years, to produce policy or environmental changes, or to observe health or social outcomes from an intervention. Identifying the most relevant measures to detect change in the short term (weeks) and medium term (months), and then utilising those measures in a correct sequence, increases the chances of detecting program effects related to the goals and objectives of an intervention. Use of a logic model (Chapter 3), and a well-developed program plan, will help to clarify what type of impact and outcome is best measured at what time in follow-up studies. It is also worth bearing in mind that some immediate effects such as program awareness or understanding may be short-lived, and are less relevant to longer term follow up, perhaps years later.

These considerations related to the timing of post-test measurement also emphasise the value of more than one follow-up study in order to detect different effects over a longer time period, and to assess whether or not short-term impact has reduced or decayed over time. As is so often the case, the inclusion of more than one follow-up study will depend very much on available funding.

The weakest design is the one group, 'post-intervention only' evaluation (type 6 in Figure 4.1). This is where people are surveyed or assessed following the program. This design should never be used for assessing program effects, as no causal inferences can be made. Such a design may only be useful for collecting process evaluation measures, such as participants' assessment of the program components or satisfaction with the program.

Using multiple designs: triangulation

This chapter has summarised the key evaluation design options, and raised some important technical issues related to the selection of populations, and the analysis and interpretation of information produced from studies. In addition to the quantitative research methods that have been the focus of the preceding sections, qualitative evaluation findings can be used to corroborate results (e.g. through an examination of information gathered through the process evaluation of implementation). Instead of arguing the relative strengths and weaknesses of quantitative/qualitative research, and experimental/ observational research, most researchers involved in the evaluation of health promotion interventions recognise the synergistic effects of combining different methods to answer the different research and evaluation questions.

One promising approach to the use of multiple methods is the concept of research 'triangulation' to improve confidence in research findings. This approach is now well established among qualitative researchers, and involves accumulating evidence from a variety of sources. The logic of this approach is that the more consistent the direction of the evidence produced from different sources, the more reasonable it is to assume that the program has produced the observed effects.

> Triangulation simply means using more than one approach to answer the same question.

Different types of triangulation can be used. For example:

- *data source triangulation*, which involves using different kinds of information to investigate a given research question, such as client records, minutes of meetings, published documents, and interviews with key informants;
- *researcher triangulation*, which involves more than one researcher in data collection and analysis—this approach

can be particularly useful if the researchers hold different theoretical and/or methodological perspectives; and

- *methods triangulation*, which involves using a number of different methods to investigate a nominated issue, such as focus group discussions, individual interviews, observation of meetings and other interactions.

The use of 'triangulation' has much merit in the evaluation of health promotion, especially where experimental research design may be inappropriate, impractical, or provide only part of the picture in a multilevel intervention. Combining information from different quantitative and qualitative sources to assess for consistency in results can provide powerful evidence of success, as well as providing insight into the processes of change in populations and organisations. It allows for consideration of observed change (or lack of change) from multiple perspectives, and offers the opportunity for confirmation of the logic of the results and the processes that produced them.

Thus, for example, in an obesity prevention study, it would strengthen the evidence demonstrating program effectiveness in reducing obesity in the community if corroborating evidence could be found, such as observable changes in healthy choices in canteens in schools and worksites, an audit of facilities that showed new physical activity facilities in the community, and, if sales of healthier foods had grown in local supermarkets compared to supermarket sales in other communities not receiving the intervention.

The generation and use of a diverse range of data and information sources will generally provide more illuminating, relevant and sensitive evidence of effects than a single source of information. Good process evaluation can be particularly important here, as it provides valuable information on how a program is implemented, what activities occur under what conditions, by whom, and with what level of effort, and will also ensure that much more is learned and understood about success or failure in achieving defined outcomes. Through this understanding it is possible to identify the conditions that need to be created to achieve successful outcomes and to reproduce these effects at different times and in different environments.

Given the different types of health promotion intervention, it will be obvious from the issues described above that there is no single approach that represents the 'best evaluation design' for all purposes.

> The 'best approach' in health promotion program evaluation will vary, depending on the context and setting of the program, the resources and time available, and the expressed needs of stakeholders for evidence of program effectiveness.

Many health promotion programs will be difficult to assess using traditional evaluation designs that are described in this chapter. In some circumstances less rigorous evaluation designs that rely more heavily on the use of information describing the process of implementation, and qualitative interpretation of observed changes in the target population, may be the only form of evaluation that is practical, and may actually be preferable to rushed, underresourced and poorly conceived impact or outcome evaluation.

Bias, sampling and data analysis

In all evaluation studies, it is essential that potential sources of bias, the sampling methods used and methods of data analysis are fully described.

Selection biases

As will be apparent from the preceding sections, in addition to the evaluation design, several important technical issues must also be addressed to ensure quality of evidence from health promotion program evaluations, and to minimise any **bias** in the results. Bias is where something differs systematically from the true situation. One source of bias that can influence the conclusions from an evaluation study concerns the characteristics of the people participating in the study, the reasons for their participation and the duration of their participation. These issues are broadly described under the heading of *selection effects*.

In considering selection effects, we need to understand how people were recruited into the study sample, and assess whether or not they were representative of the people in the whole population or community. For example, if volunteers enrol in a study, then they are likely to be more motivated and/or have higher health literacy than people who did not volunteer. This will probably exaggerate the results from an intervention, as motivated volunteers, better educated and socially confident individuals would typically respond more positively to health promotion interventions. This would result in better outcomes than would be observed if the program was delivered to a more representative population that may contain motivated and unmotivated people. This source of bias is especially important where a program is intended to have greatest impact among more marginalised or disadvantaged populations who may be harder to contact, and less motivated to participate. This commonly occurs in health promotion interventions, and is a good reason for subsequent replication studies to assess if the initial study effects are generalisable to other settings.

Selection bias may also occur as a consequence of a person selected to participate in a study refusing to do so (**non-response bias**). Again, in such circumstances those who agree to participate in a study may be different from those who do not agree to participate, resulting in different effects than would be observed if the program were delivered to a fully representative population. For example, if an intervention to improve prevention counselling in primary care was targeted at 200 primary care physicians and only obtains 20 participants (as 180 refused), the effects of counselling from these 20 could not be considered as reflecting the effectiveness of physicians in general for this intervention.

In both cases, if the people in the study are not similar to the whole population, then the results of the study may not be **generalisable**—they cannot be extrapolated to the whole population. In these circumstances, even a large and statistically significant result from a study must be treated with caution, as the population effects could not be assumed to be the same.

A further source of bias concerns *subject retention*—that is, how many people who start a program actually finish it. This may be a source of bias if those who drop out of a program are different in their characteristics and behaviours from those who complete a program.

Similarly, if a person participates in a pretest study, but is unable to be contacted or refuses to participate in a post-test study, this too may be a source of bias if the population participating in the pretest study is different from the population that participates in the post-test study. The extent of **drop out** or **loss to follow up** influences the usefulness of the findings, and the results of the study may not be generalisable.

For these reasons, it is not only important to do everything that is practically possible to obtain a representative sample, but also important to maintain a high participation rate throughout the study. Maintaining people in evaluation studies may require the use of simple-to-complete questionnaires, active communication with and encouragement of study subjects, and sometimes the provision of incentives for continued participation. Further issues related to questionnaire design are considered in Chapter 5. Importantly, the impact of selection bias, and non-response bias, need to be described and considered for their influence on results in any report of an evaluation.

Sampling methods

In small-scale interventions, we may be able to measure everyone who is targeted for intervention. In large community-wide programs that are intended to reach thousands of people, this is not practical, nor is it needed for the purposes of evaluation. In such circumstances we can rely upon a **sample** of a subset of individuals from the population to assess the impact of the program. The way in which we recruit people to small-scale studies and the way in which we sample them for the evaluation of large studies are also important for the generalisability of the findings. By using a **random sample**, the effects of the program can be considered applicable to the whole source population. Random sampling implies that a list of the whole population that is targeted by an intervention exists, and that it is possible to select subjects for an evaluation study at random (i.e. each person has an equal chance of being selected or not being selected).

Examples of such population-level lists include census lists, health clinic or health insurance lists, employee payroll lists, lists of populations of patients registered in primary care, school lists of enrolled pupils and telephone listings (where there is very high telephone ownership).

In some cases, it will not be possible or practical to achieve a true random sample from a population, especially in a situation where no population 'list' or record exists from which to select a random sample (e.g. among homeless people or other highly marginalised groups). In this case, one of the alternative methods in Table 4.1 should be attempted. Table 4.1 uses two examples to illustrate different types of sampling that can be used in evaluation studies.

Statistics and the analysis of data

A serious examination of biostatistics is well beyond the scope of this book, but an understanding of basic statistical concepts is needed during the planning phase of a program, and for the critical appraisal

Table 4.1 Sampling and recruitment methods applied to the evaluation of large-scale and small-scale interventions

	Recruitment of participants to a small health promotion trial[1]	Sampling of people to evaluate a large-scale intervention[2]
Best sampling methods providing generalisable results	Random sampling from the population of people with chronic arthritis	Random sample of women aged 50–59 is measured—sampling of the at-risk whole population allows every individual an equal chance of selection
	Sampling from a defined database of people with arthritis	
	Sampling from numerous community groups and clinic settings—even if non-random, may show enough diversity to be generalisable	Other variants: random sampling with increased samples (oversampling) of specific groups of interest, such as an ethnic group who is less likely to be screened; sometimes if the population is small, survey everybody (known as a 'universal sample')
	Snowball samples, where hard-to-reach groups can be found through social networks—this has the potential to produce reasonable samples	
Less useful sampling methods providing less reliable results	Volunteers with arthritis recruited through newspaper advertisements, or through arthritis clinics in the local hospital	Non-random (convenient) sampling: street intercept samples; other convenient samples from women attending a group or club or belonging to an organisation

1 for example, a trial of an education program to increase patient confidence in the self-management of chronic arthritis
2 for example, a community education program to increase the rate of mammography screening for all women aged 50–59

of other people's evaluation studies. Further reading is recommended at the end of this chapter.

The **sample size calculation** is used to determine how many people are needed for an evaluation study. For example, an obesity prevention program might determine an objective for the intervention community to lose an average of 3 kg of weight over 12 months. With known measures (and with an understanding of their variation), it is possible to calculate the number of people who will need to be measured to detect an effect of a prespecified size. This should be estimated before the evaluation starts. The sample size is also related to the statistical *power* of the study which, put simply, is the probability of detecting a difference between the intervention and the control groups.

> Ultimately, no matter how good the quality of the data collected, if it is not analysed and interpreted well, it will not produce useful information on the success or otherwise of an intervention.

To this end, we have to consider the use of statistical methods to analyse and make sense of quantitative information gathered through quantitative evaluation studies.

One key analytical technique is to determine the **statistical significance** of a result—to determine whether the results observed might have occurred by chance. This is referred to as the level of statistical significance. Statistical significance describes the probability of the observed results (i.e. the difference in a target outcome when comparing the measure before and after an intervention, and/or between intervention and control groups) occurring by chance. Statistical significance is often described using terms such as p values, which are often described in published papers as <0.05 or <0.01. This simply means that there is a 1 in 20, or 1 in 100, possibility of an observed outcome occurring by chance, respectively.

Another related statistical concept is the use of **confidence intervals** around an observed outcome. In this case, confidence intervals describe how likely are the true population results to be outside of the range described by the confidence limits.

Other statistical tests require consideration of the type and distribution of the data collected—specifically, whether data is a 'continuous' measure (e.g. the number of cigarettes smoked each day), or is the outcome just described as a category (improved/did not improve; or smoker/nonsmoker). Different statistical tests are required for continuous data (these include parametric tests, such as *t* tests and Pearson correlation coefficients), compared to data in categories (such as chi-squared statistics, and odds ratios).

Finally, in analysing the results from an evaluation, consideration has to be given to whether the results observed might be due to some other factors, either in the data, or external to the program. This is usually referred to as a **confounder**. Internal factors might contribute in subtle ways. It may be that one group improves most because it is more socially connected or has greater confidence about achieving the outcomes. External factors might contribute to changes in outcomes in both intervention and control groups; these factors could be national or global background trends. For example, in many countries, tobacco use has declined and community views on restricting smoking in indoor environments have strengthened. A health promotion program in a defined community to address these issues would have to consider the rate of background changes, and assess whether their program could produce effects greater than these existing **secular trends**.

Similarly, the background effects of large-scale national programs (such as media campaigns) may reduce or confuse the effect of a local-level program. For example, the impact of a national media campaign to promote uptake of immunisation against influenza among older people might completely mask the impact of a more local campaign by a health clinic to improve uptake. It is also worth recognising that it may not always be positive change that indicates program success. For example, given the increases in obesity in many countries, a local program that demonstrated no change in obesity prevalence over five years at the same time as national prevalence was rising would be a success. In such circumstances, having a control region, or national serial monitoring data as 'normative control', would be essential, and allow this intervention to be appraised as a successful innovation.

As we have stressed before, it is essential that these sources of bias, the sampling methods used, and methods of data analysis are fully described in any report on an evaluation study.

Evaluation designs for health promotion replication and dissemination

The previous section described the evaluation of individual interventions, identifying the key evaluation design options, and summarising some important technical issues. Through such an evaluation process, some health promotion interventions would have been found to be effective, affordable and well implemented; others would not meet these criteria. Once a program is shown to be effective in certain settings, we need to know whether the program works as well and in the same ways in other settings and environments. This is the fourth stage in Figure 2.1, intervention demonstration (program replication).

Intervention demonstration (replication)

There are several purposes for conducting replication or demonstration studies. Repeated findings of intervention effects assist health authorities and program funders in identifying programs suitable for adoption, policy support and wide-scale **dissemination**. Alternatively, it is risky and unwise to base a decision to scale up a program and commit significant funding on the basis of one evaluation study at one point in time in one setting.

The first purpose of replication is to confirm the scientific findings of program effectiveness, and to assess whether similar effects are found when the study is repeated in similar populations. This is important, because the effects observed in the original study may not be repeated, as they may have been due to specific characteristics in the samples used in the initial study, the level of enthusiasm or commitment of stakeholders, or unique characteristics of the setting in which the initial evaluation was conducted. Replication increases confidence that the effects are real, and that this level of change in short-term and long-term outcomes might be achieved elsewhere.

The second purpose of replication studies is to assess the generalisability of the effects produced in different populations and settings. Often the initial study effects were seen on volunteers, motivated people, or socially and educationally advantaged groups of high health literacy. It is important to demonstrate how well the program works when it is tested among people from different socioeconomic groups and diverse cultural backgrounds. The number of replications is not fixed; this depends on the policy priorities in the region or country, but at least one replication of a program in a different setting is a minimal standard.

Finally, and most importantly, the process of replication assists in understanding the processes of implementing a program in different settings.

These reasons for further study before widespread dissemination become more obvious when individual effectiveness studies are examined more closely. For example, Figure 4.3 shows a hypothetical community with 35 worksites. A comprehensive worksite health promotion program might have been tested with four worksites, marked with an X, and shown to be effective in producing a range of outcomes among individual workers in intervention when compared to workers in control sites. What may not be so evident from the study results is that the worksite contained a much higher proportion of white-collar workers, and that the management were highly supportive of the program implementation.

In such circumstances, it is essential to examine whether these same effects would be found in other worksites, marked as Y in the figure. These worksites might be different from those enrolled in the original trial. Specific worksites might be chosen for the further testing of the intervention—some to be similar, and some quite different, such as worksites with a higher proportion of blue-collar workers, or worksites with different age/gender distributions or less obvious management support.

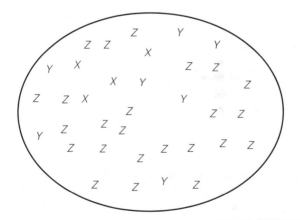

Legend
X = worksites in original trial
Y = worksites in replication
Z = all other worksites in region

Figure 4.3 Replication and dissemination in worksites in a defined geographical area

The research methods in this phase are directed to two central goals:

- Can the *program effects be replicated* in similar and in dissimilar settings, or will the effect sizes for individual-level and organisational-level outcomes vary?
- Can the *program implementation be replicated* in diverse settings?

The first research aim requires further evaluation using the same outcome measures. Here, it would be determined if the effects produced in the original trial were typical by assessing whether a program run in a worksite with different characteristics or population mix, or with a different level of management support, produces similar changes at the individual and organisational level.

The evaluation designs here could replicate the earlier designs, such as the quasi-experimental design with control groups, or could just be a 'before–after' design in the individual Y worksites. The reason why the latter design is acceptable here is that the effect size (i.e. the change in the target outcomes) is already known, estimated from the original trial. Hence, even 'before–after' designs in single new worksites will provide a useful demonstration of program effects, and will allow estimation of the effects in these individual replicate settings. The worksites for replication would not need to be randomly chosen. Indeed, in replication studies purposive sampling to maximise the diversity of settings for examination would be most useful.

The second research aim is concerned with process evaluation in these Y sites. The major task of intervention demonstration is to show that the program can be implemented in the ways intended in different settings.

> Testing the implementation in diverse and real-world settings is considered an essential prerequisite before population-level dissemination.

For example, the original trial might have had a worker consultation committee, management support, and a budget for internal social marketing. These elements might have been shown as necessary for positive outcomes in the original trial, and the replication study would test whether these different intervention elements could be reproduced. This process evaluation across sites is a core element at this stage of the development of an intervention, providing further essential information on the circumstances under which the original outcomes could be reproduced. This type of information is essential for health practitioners who have responsibility for implementing programs, because if these proven elements cannot be replicated in these demonstration sites, then further implementation of the program in different sites would not yield the same results as the original program.

If the program implementation proves possible in a range of sites, and the intervention effect is maintained, then this program is considered feasible for more widespread distribution within the whole community.

Dissemination and institutionalisation

Initial program evaluation and replication studies demonstrate whether an intervention works, the magnitude of effects expected, and whether it works to the same degree in different settings. If a program has demonstrated public-health effects in different contexts and settings, it may be considered worthy of wider dissemination across systems, regions or indeed across a whole country. At this stage, we need to consider the ways in which an effective program might be disseminated to reach the whole target population.

This next step, intervention dissemination (stage 5 in Figure 2.1), is an active and intentional process of achieving the maximum uptake of effective and feasible interventions into a community. There are several stages in diffusion, but the aim is to introduce effective interventions into the majority of target sites, shown as 'Z' in Figure 4.3, who have not been engaged in any of the testing or demonstration phases of evaluation.

Effective dissemination depends upon original evidence of effectiveness (stage 3 effectiveness studies), evidence of adaptable implementation in diverse situations (stage 4 replication studies), and will need continuing commitment from decision makers and program funders. This latter requirement may produce supportive policy to enable the distribution of the program, and may provide resources or support to enable the widespread uptake of the program across a community.

Evaluation tasks at this phase are more strongly focused on process evaluation, particularly in examining factors affecting uptake, and the sustainability of the program. One example of a research study of the dissemination process in health promotion is provided by the

CATCH program in the USA (see Box 4.4). In this example, successful dissemination was found to be dependent upon a number of elements that offer general guidance on what needs to be examined and assessed in a dissemination study. These include:

- *Assessment of uptake.* Who participates and who does not, and what are the reasons? This involves process evaluation, and comparisons of attributes of participants and non-participants.

- *Assessing consistency in the application of program intervention elements.* How much local variation and adaptation takes place? In the CATCH example, this variation was minimised by standardisation of the program materials. This involves process evaluation, monitoring the program elements against a standardised approach, and assessing how and where the program implementation deviates from the initial trial.

- *Assessment of the 'political engagement' of key individuals and organisations that might facilitate or block successful implementation, and understanding the reasons for different levels of engagement.* In the CATCH example, these were the school boards and school principals. Evaluation here comprises ongoing process measures of commitment and participation by these stakeholders; this could include quantitative or qualitative methods.

- *Assessing the engagement and training of the key program implementers to understand variation in uptake and implementation at the point of delivery.* In the CATCH example, a majority of teachers who were responsible for 'delivering' key elements of the intervention were engaged in a training program to improve motivation and consistency of delivery. Again this is process evaluation; here 'quality control' of the intervention would be ascertained by teacher surveys or direct observations, to ensure that teachers trained in diverse settings were delivering an overall program consistent with the CATCH approach.

Other evaluation tasks in program dissemination are to document the costs, staffing required, presence of consistent planning approaches (logic models) in each setting, and developing tools for continuous tracking and monitoring.

Box 4.4 Case study: dissemination of the CATCH program

The CATCH program (Hoelscher et al., 2001), initially known as the 'Child and Adolescent Trial for Cardiovascular Health', was initially evaluated as a cluster RCT among 96 schools across the USA, among late-primary-school-age children. The project had good formative and process evaluation (McGraw et al., 1994). The impact of the intervention showed it to be effective, especially in improving on primary school nutrition and physical activity patterns, as well as on school climate (Luepker et al., 1996).

Two efforts at dissemination have been reported, both in Texas (Heath and Coleman, 2003; Hoelscher et al., 2001). Both reported that the curricula materials had been standardised for broader use and that, through working with school boards, obtaining resources and adopting a proactive model for dissemination, the CATCH program (which had changed its name to the more generic 'A Coordinated Approach to Child Health') had been successfully disseminated to over 700 schools in three-quarters of all the school boards in Texas, and had trained teachers from 528 of these schools. Further successful dissemination has occurred since this publication.

However, the successful dissemination and adoption of the program did not imply usage by all enrolled schools, and ongoing monitoring of the process in all new sites was considered an essential evaluation element.

The last stage in the program development and evaluation process (stage 6 in Figure 2.1)—program monitoring—concerns the monitoring of a program that has been widely disseminated, and is routinely implemented. This stage of evaluation is primarily concerned with quality control and long-term monitoring and surveillance of outcomes at a population level. This applies in a situation where a program has been successfully diffused into a community, has established policy support and funding mechanisms, and has continuing community support. At this stage, the project is becoming institutionalised (i.e. **institutionalisation**), and is integrated into the long-term functions of the host agency or organisation. The evaluation tasks are:

- regular population monitoring to assess maintenance of behaviours, beliefs or understanding;
- monitoring of community engagement with the project, support for the project, and community capacity that may result from the project;
- process evaluation/quality control of the delivery of programs across the community; and
- process monitoring of policy and environmental changes, their adherence and implementation as planned.

The basis for evaluation of institutionalised programs is through routine population surveillance. In many regions, there are representative sample health surveys, to which specific health promotion questions can be added. These surveys monitor trends in community beliefs and perceptions towards health issues, as well as health behaviours. In the worksite example above, annual population surveys of working-age adults might show increased opinions that healthy food choices are important, stronger support for smoke-free areas in workplaces, and changes in dietary behaviour among individuals. Trend data can be accumulated to demonstrate population effects over time, or to demonstrate a reversal in program effects if the program's hold or reach weakens, and program adherence declines over time.

This information is acquired in the background, and is linked to routine surveys, not specifically conducted for monitoring the institutionalisation of this program. This set of research tasks is also relevant for monitoring the implementation of national programs or initiatives and health promotion guidelines. National-level surveys can be used to monitor these outcomes over time.

The second component is the monitoring of representative or leading community stakeholders, coalitions and taskforces, to assess their ongoing support for the program (Reger-Nash et al., 2006). This can be in the form of surveys, qualitative interviews or policy analysis to assess the progress towards institutional acceptance and implementation from a decision-maker and resource-allocation perspective.

Process evaluation remains central in stage 6 evaluation, and will require some resources and effort. Implementation across many sites requires quality control, to make sure that the programs delivered have enough elements of the original program to still be effective. These evaluation tasks can assist decision makers in the ongoing maintenance of established programs. Box 4.5 lists a range of examples of the type of research question that could be addressed in this evaluation phase.

Box 4.5 Examples of policy and environmental evaluation tasks for institutionalised programs

Monitoring of health service and other sector program delivery

- Are established physical education (PE) programs continuing to be delivered by the education sector to all schools?
- Do established needle and syringe exchange programs continue to be widely available in the health system? In outreach clinics or environments?
- Are ongoing cancer screening services accessed by all target population groups?
- Do drug and alcohol programs reach all marginalised youth?
- Are self-management programs for chronic illness available to all eligible individuals (e.g. asthma education programs, cardiac rehabilitation programs)?

Monitoring of policy: maintenance and adherence in the community

- Is a policy (e.g. restricting tobacco sales to minors) being adhered to by merchants of small stores near schools?
- Are policies about advertising of unhealthy foods to children being adhered to?
- Are urban development policies with a health impact being complied with?
- As part of an institutionalised 'safe sex' campaign, are condoms freely available from a range of outlets in the community?

Summary

This chapter has focused on the different evaluation tasks and designs needed to test effectiveness, and replicate and disseminate health promotion programs. In testing innovative interventions, careful attention to evaluation design is needed, as is a good understanding of several important technical issues related to the selection of populations, and the analysis and interpretation of information produced from studies. The better the evaluation design and methods that we use in assessing impact and outcome, the more confident we can be that the observed effects of a program were caused by the intervention and did not occur by chance, or were not due to other factors or influences.

> Experimental designs that are built on successful completion of the health promotion intervention as planned, and use large and representative samples of the study population and valid measures before and after the intervention, offer the best evidence of effectiveness.

As emphasised in Chapter 3, careful and systematic process evaluation provides the foundation on which effectiveness can be assessed, as well as providing valuable insight on the practicalities of implementation. This knowledge is essential for subsequent replication and dissemination studies. Information from process evaluation is also invaluable in interpreting the impact of evaluation data and its likely causal link to the program.

We have emphasised that the diversity of settings and complexity of interventions often mean that it is not possible to evaluate health promotion programs using experimental/RCT designs. Alternative designs, especially quasi-experimental designs, may be the most feasible in many situations. Other designs that rely more heavily on the use of information describing the process of implementation, and qualitative interpretation of data, may be less methodologically rigorous, but may actually be preferable to rushed, underresourced and poorly conceived experimental designs.

We have also stressed that the generation and use of a diverse range of data and information sources will generally provide more illuminating, relevant and sensitive evidence of effects than a single source of information. Process evaluation not only provides valuable information on how a program is implemented, what activities occur under what conditions, by whom, and with what level of effort, but will also ensure that much more is learned and understood about success or failure in achieving defined outcomes. Through this understanding, it is possible to identify the conditions that need to be created to achieve successful outcomes and to reproduce these effects at different times and in different environments.

'Best practice' in health promotion evaluation will always require consideration of the 'optimal against the possible' in evaluation design. There is no single approach that represents the best evaluation design for all purposes. The best approach in health promotion program evaluation will vary, depending on the context and setting of the program, the resources and time available, and the expressed needs of stakeholders for evidence of program effectiveness.

Finally, once an intervention has been demonstrated to be effective, the evaluation task is not over. The intervention should be replicated in other settings, and, if it maintains effectiveness in different environments, it should be disseminated. In these latter stages, process evaluation, often using qualitative research methods, is the most important component, to ensure that the program is delivered across a community in ways likely to maintain effectiveness. Finally, as programs become institutionalised, population surveys can be used to track outcomes, and continuing process evaluation used to ensure quality control across larger regions or national program rollout. Thus, evaluation tasks start with individual trials, but continue on to assess the extent to which the whole target group can access and participate in the program on a continuing basis, and that the program is contributing to population-level health gain.

In all evaluation studies, it is essential that the evaluation design and research methods are well described. This includes an obligation to fully describe potential sources of bias, the sampling methods used, and methods of data analysis in any report on an evaluation study.

References

DiClemente, R.J., Wingood, G.M., Harrington, K.F., Lang, D.L., Davies, S.L., Hook, E.W. 3rd et al. (2004), 'Efficacy of an HIV Prevention Intervention for African American Adolescent Girls: A Randomized Controlled Trial', *JAMA*, 292(2), pp. 171–9.

Forster, J., Murray, D.M., Wolfson, M., Blaine, T., Wagenaar, A., Hennrikus, D. (1998), 'The Effects of Community Policies to Reduce Youth Access to Tobacco', *American Journal of Public Health*, 88, pp. 1193–8.

Heath, E.M., Coleman, K.J. (2003), 'Adoption and Institutionalization of the Child and Adolescent Trial for Cardiovascular Health (CATCH) in El Paso, Texas', *Health Promotion Practice*, 4(2), pp. 157–64.

Hoelscher, D.M., Kelder, S.H., Murray, N., Cribb, P.W. (2001), 'Dissemination and Adoption of the Child and Adolescent Trial for Cardiovascular Health (CATCH): A Case Study in Texas', *Journal of Public Health Management and Practice*, 7(2), pp. 90–100.

Luepker, R.V., Perry, C.L., McKinlay, S.M., Nader, P.R., Parcel, G.S., Stone, E.J. et al. (1996), 'Outcomes of a Field Trial to Improve Children's Dietary Patterns and Physical Activity: The Child and Adolescent Trial for Cardiovascular Health. CATCH "Collaborative Group"', *JAMA*, 275(10), pp. 768–76.

McGraw, S.A., Stone, E.J., Osganian, S.K., Elder, J.P., Perry, C.L., Johnson, C.C. et al. (1994), 'Design of Process Evaluation within the Child and Adolescent Trial for Cardiovascular Health (CATCH)', *Health Education Quarterly*, Suppl 2, s5–s26.

Reger, W., Cooper, L., Butterfield-Booth, S., Bauman, A. (2002), 'Wheeling Walks: A Community Campaign Using Paid Media to Encourage Walking Among Sedentary Older Adults', *Preventive Medicine*, September, pp. 285–92.

Reger-Nash, B., Bauman, A., Cooper, L., Chey, T., Simon, K. (in press, 2006), *Evaluating Community Wide Walking Interventions. Evaluation and Program Planning*.

Shelley, J.M., Irwig, L.M., Simpson, J.M., Macaskill, P. (1991), 'Evaluation of a Mass-Media-Led Campaign to Increase Pap Smear Screening', *Health Education Research*, 6(3), pp. 267–77.

Further reading

Elwood, J.M. (1998), *Critical Appraisal of Epidemiological Studies and Clinical Trials*, Oxford University Press, Oxford.

Flay, B.R., Biglan, A., Boruch, R.F. (2005), 'Standards of Evidence: Criteria for Efficacy, Effectiveness and Dissemination', *Prevention Science*, September, pp. 1–25.

Florey, C. (1993), 'Sample Size for Beginners', *British Medical Journal*, 306, pp. 1181–4.

Green, L.W., Lewis, F.M. (1986), *Measurement and Evaluation in Health Education and Health Promotion*, Mayfield Publishing Company, Mountain View, California.

Chapter 5
Measurement in health promotion programs

Purpose of health promotion measurement

Chapter 4 identified several technical challenges in the evaluation of health promotion interventions. These included sampling, data analysis and the measurement of outcomes. This chapter provides a more detailed examination of the principles and practicalities of measurement in health promotion, with special reference to program evaluation.

A fundamental component of any organised effort to promote health is the accurate and consistent measurement of the outcomes. Health promotion measurements should enable us to:

- describe the magnitude of health problems in individuals, groups or communities, as a part of the planning of an intervention;
- assess the impact and effectiveness of health promotion programs, by detecting changes in outcomes, including assessing changes in the intermediate and short-term outcome measures described in Chapter 1;
- explain how health promotion programs work, through an understanding of the **determinants** and **correlates** of health promotion outcomes during a program—that is, through measurement of process or intermediate **variables**, and assessment of the relationship between these and program outcomes; and
- routinely monitor progress in health promotion outcomes at the population level.

This chapter provides an overview of some of the technical challenges that have to be addressed to achieve these goals.

Modes of measurement and data collection

Some attributes or characteristics that we want to measure in health promotion are directly observable. For example, height and weight (obesity measures), blood pressure or serum cholesterol levels can be assessed through direct measurement. These may be relevant to health promotion programs, as impact or health outcome measures. These are described as 'objective' measurements or **observable phenomena**.

Others are not so directly observable—knowledge, attitudes, public opinion and even most health behaviours cannot be directly measured in the same way as the physical and biological markers referred to above. These are referred to as **non-observable phenomena** and have to be indirectly assessed (e.g. through surveys that are self-completed, or questions that are asked through face-to-face or telephone interviews).

The definition and measurement of intermediate health outcomes, such as health behaviours and healthy environments, and the health promotion outcomes that may influence them, has taxed the skills of researchers for decades. The task may be relatively straightforward in the case of defining and measuring smoking behaviour using information provided by individuals, but more complex in other areas such as assessing dietary behaviour or patterns of physical activity. Measuring knowledge, attitudes or values, personal and social skills as indicators of health literacy, public opinion and community competency as measures of social mobilisation, and organisational and environmental change, are even more problematical.

The solution to many of the problems of measurement is found in the construction of questionnaires, tests and scales (mostly self-administered by individuals), as well as face-to-face interview protocols that can produce both quantitative and qualitative information. Such research tools not only are used to obtain information from individuals on personal knowledge, attitudes and behaviours, but also can be used to obtain information from relevant respondents on organisational policy and practice, and on community capacity and competence.

It is not possible to consider in detail the process of constructing this type of research tool—whole books are written on this subject, and some are recommended at the end of the chapter. However, there are several important technical concepts that need to be understood by the critical practitioner, and these are considered below.

Reliability, validity and responsiveness

Key elements of any measurement are that they are reliable and valid. **Reliability** refers to the stability of a measure—assessing the extent to which each time the measure is used, and for each person it is used with, it will measure the same thing. This is relatively straightforward when asking a person a simple factual question, such as where they live. However, it is much less simple when attempting to assess self-confidence (e.g. in refusing an alcoholic drink). In this latter example, a more complex set of information is required, some of which is subjective to the individual.

The most common method used to test and develop reliability is to repeat administration of the measurement on the same subject using the same administration procedures within a short period of time to see if this *test–retest* procedure produces the same results. This is also described as 'repeatability' of measurement. Thus, in the example above, if the same subject answers a set of questions on self-efficacy in relation to a specific task in the same way within a relatively short period of time, the measurement can be considered stable and reliable.

Testing for reliability is important even when the object of study can be observed directly (e.g. observing and rating the characteristics of an environment, such as a house or a school). In this case, reliability can be determined by the level of agreement between two observers or 'raters' of the same phenomenon. This is known as *interrater reliability*. This is important where different people are assessing the same thing (e.g. where a group of researchers is making observations on similar environments). If the recorded observations differed too much, then the measurement would be unreliable. In such a case, strict guidelines would need to be developed for the way in which data is collected by researchers to minimise variations in observation, and/or the number of observers could be reduced to minimise the likelihood of variation.

Validity is the assessment of the 'truth' of a measurement. A question, scale or test is considered *valid* to the extent it measures what it intended to measure. A reliable measurement is not necessarily a valid measurement—you may be measuring the wrong thing, but doing so consistently.

One of the most commonly advocated approaches to assessment of validity is the use of biochemical or physiological tests, where these tests are considered 'true' measures of the factors of interest (e.g. the measurement of cotinine in a saliva or blood sample to detect recent tobacco use as a test of validity of self-reported smoking behaviour, the measurement of blood lipids to validate aspects of self-reported diet, the measurement of serum antibodies to validate immunisation status, and so on). Although desirable, such measures are generally difficult and expensive, and not always practical to use. Generally, such objective validation is only available to support measures of behaviour. Measurement of attitudes and beliefs, and psychosocial concepts like self-efficacy, do not offer themselves to such objective validation, and the development of valid measurements has proved to be a challenging task for researchers.

Initial simple procedures can be employed to check that a measurement has **face validity** and **content validity**. The concept of *face validity* is that experts in the field think the measure is a useful way of assessing the dimension of interest. The concept of *content validity* is that the items cover all of the areas expected for the measure.

In order to optimise measurement properties, a question, scale or test should present options to a subject in a balanced way and one that allows the respondent to answer across the full range of potential responses. This can be achieved, for example, by asking someone the extent to which they agree or disagree with a statement such as 'I think that smoking should be banned in all indoor areas'. The options for response to such a question can be refined by offering different potential responses in the form of a ranked scale, such as 'agree strongly', 'agree', 'neither agree nor disagree', 'disagree', 'disagree strongly'. This form of question design is referred to as a **Likert scale**. A person replying to this type of question is able to express their answer in different degrees, and the evaluator is able to analyse the differences in response to the question in a more sophisticated way. Some of the more commonly used elements of questionnaire design are described below.

More complex is the challenge to develop valid measures of concepts such as 'social capital', or 'capacity building', where the constituent elements of the concept are not agreed by experts. This depends upon an understanding of the relationship between **concepts**, **variables** and **constructs**. A *concept* is an organising idea, often theoretical, used to describe a phenomenon that is not directly observable. In health promotion we use concepts such as community capacity, self-efficacy and social influence on a regular basis. These concepts are not directly observable, but are important elements in the development and implementation of a health promotion intervention, and form elements of the impact and outcome of programs.

The process of taking these concepts or ideas, and turning them into actual measures (**levels of measurement**), is a technical and sometimes complex process derived from psychology and other social sciences. The objective is to turn concepts into *variables*, which are validly and reliably measurable, and, as the name suggests, capable of showing variation between subjects, and variation as a consequence of intervention (responsive). Variables may be single *items*, or summarised as composite **scales** or **scores**.

For example, there is no direct method for observing 'community capacity' or 'social influence'. These *concepts* can be described, and questions (single-item variables) generated, which are thought to be related to them. These questions can then be administered to people in a defined population group. Once data is available from a population, psychometric statistical techniques, derived from psychology and other social sciences, can be used to describe the measurement properties of these underlying constructs, and to describe how well the items are related to the construct—in other words, to describe, statistically, how well the construct 'exists'. This is called *construct validation*.

The steps in the development of a measure and its quantitative testing are shown in Box 5.1 on page 92. This describes a set of logical steps for those developing measures. The statistical procedures mentioned here are referred to in this chapter and in Chapter 4. For those developing and validating their own measures, this box provides a checklist for the stages in measurement development. However, in many circumstances, the wisest option is to identify, understand and use relevant measures developed by others.

To help understand the strengths and weaknesses of different types of measure, Table 5.1 provides examples of the methods used in reliability and validity studies in health promotion, and the statistical methods that will be encountered in measurement studies. The purpose here is for readers to become familiar with the names of these statistical tests and understand the context and purposes for which the test is used. Examples chosen are from health-promotion-relevant measurement development. Note that many measurement studies report test–retest repeatability, **internal consistency** of scales or scores, and construct validity in the same paper. Table 5.1 describes the differences between these procedures and their use in health promotion measurement development and testing. Further reading or consultation with an expert in measurement (a psychometrician) and/or statistician is recommended before their use.

Table 5.1 Statistical techniques used to test for reliability and validity

Type of reliability or validity	Typical statistical methods used	Example from a health promotion measurement study: purpose of the measurement development	Examples of the statistics/coefficients used for measurement development purposes in the study
Reliability			
Test–retest repeatability	Usually *intraclass* correlation (ICC); sometimes *Spearman's rho* for non-parametric data (skewed distributions). For categorical data (data in two or a few categories) the *kappa* coefficient is often used (weighted kappa if more than two categories)	Brown and colleagues (2004) tested the reliability of four different physical activity survey questionnaires in a population sample in order to assess which was more reliable, and which components of the questionnaires were most reliable	Four self-report instruments were compared, and were administered twice on serial days to the same people. Per cent agreement for the proportions 'sufficiently active' ranged from 0.6 to 0.8, but, adjusted for chance, kappa coefficients were 0.4 to 0.52 (moderate reliability). ICC values showed that walking and vigorous physical activity questions were more reliable than moderate-intensity physical activity questions. The study showed national policy makers that the existing survey questions were more reliable in the Australian context than newer international measures
Inter-rater reliability	Assessing two raters to measure agreement (usually, ICC or kappa coefficient are used)	Ademiluyi et al. (2003) developed three tools for assessing the quality of internet-based health promotion materials on smoking cessation. These three scales were each assessed by two raters	This could be important in the formative development of a program; how well do different raters agree in scoring the quality of health promotion resources? The individual items in the three scales were scored by two independent raters; for scale 1, nine of the 21 items showed reasonably good agreement between raters (kappa value >0.6), but for scale 2 only one of seven items showed this level of agreement, and for scale 3, only two of 16 items showed a kappa value of >0.6. These kappa values are for assessing agreement in categorical questions. If we compute a total score for the first scale (by summing the 21 items), then we have a continuous score and the agreement can be assessed using the ICC (in this paper for the total scale 1, the ICC was moderate at 0.54)

Table 5.1 Statistical techniques used to test for reliability and validity *(cont.)*

Type of reliability or validity	Typical statistical methods used	Example from a health promotion measurement study: purpose of the measurement development	Examples of the statistics/coefficients used for measurement development purposes in the study
Reliability (cont.)			
Responsiveness	This is testing the measurement's capacity to respond in an effective program; thus, use of the usual analytic methods would be used to assess statistical significance, such as a *t* test (if continuous data) or an odds ratio (if categorical)	This is the same thing as measuring change following a program—the outcome used needs to show measurable change in response to an effective intervention; there are no specific examples in the literature, but a good example would show significant changes in intervention groups and limited or no change in controls (see Figure 5.2)	Standard tests for significance of observed differences; all the usual statistical tests might be used to demonstrate responsiveness (*t* tests, non-parametric tests, chi-squared tests, odds ratios with 95% confidence intervals)
Validity			
Cronbach's alpha coefficient	Not a statistical test; related to number of items and mean inter-item correlation; is a measure of how well a group of items reflects an underlying construct (often thought of as a form of internal consistency of items, and classified under reliability): *Cronbach's alpha* is used for ordinal data (categories); where there are only two categories, the KR-20 coefficient is used	Barrett et al. (2005) developed scales to measure health promotion leadership at the organisational level in a Canadian region. The study closely followed all of the measurement development steps suggested in Box 5.1 (but this focuses on how Cronbach's alpha was used)	The questions were developed and tested with experts (content and face validity) and then refined and piloted. Psychometric testing (using factor analysis techniques) defined four underlying dimensions (constructs) of health promotion leadership; these four subscales were: 1 organisational learning; 2 wellness planning; 3 workplace environment; and 4 professional development. Each of these subscales was tested for internal consistency—how well did the constituent items correlate with each subscale, as measured by Cronbach's alpha values (0.91, 0.86, 0.79 and 0.80 respectively)? These subscales were deemed internally consistent
Construct validity	Whether the score or scale measures an underlying non-observed theoretical construct; usually demonstrated through data reduction techniques, such as *exploratory factor analysis*, or, when testing theoretical structure, using *confirmatory factor analysis* to see how well the data fit the theory	De Guia et al. (2003) surveyed 553 Canadian policy makers regarding their views underpinning tobacco legislation; the authors hypothesised *a priori* that there would be three underlying dimensions; the questions asked about tobacco policy—that makers thought about tobacco policy—which: 1 affected voters in the community; 2 affected the tobacco industry; and 3 influenced other community groups	Using *confirmatory factor analysis*, the analysis demonstrated the strong existence of these underlying dimensions (factors) in the questions asked; the data showed a good fit in the statistical model. Further, compared to external hypothesised criteria (this is criterion validity), they showed that non-smokers had more favourable mean attitude scores on these three factors compared to smokers (as predicted)

Box 5.1 Stages in scale or score development

1. Identify items (questions) that reflect the idea or concept of the measurement; then generate a comprehensive pool of questions that covers all the dimensions (*content validity*).
2. Test the questions with experts. Do a range of experts think these are comprehensive questions and cover the areas of importance (*face validity*, opinion of experts)?
3. Test in a sample of the target population (**pilot testing** of measures, often using only a small sample size; test qualitatively using focus groups or interviews to ascertain views about the questions, as well as testing quantitatively, and look at the distribution of responses to the questions; it is better if there is a spread of responses).
4. Reduce those with poor *item–total correlation* (e.g. using Cronbach's alpha coefficient). This means reducing the total number of questions (*data reduction*).
5. Construct subscales, using *exploratory or confirmatory factor analysis* or other methods, to further reduce the number of items. Develop underlying 'constructs' of groups of questions. These form the scales or subscales that are the 'composite measures' of the dimensions proposed.

Finally, the purpose of a health promotion intervention is to produce change related to predetermined goals and objectives. To this end a measure should also be capable of changing in response to an intervention. This is known as measurement **responsiveness**. Again, this is relatively easy when measuring a discrete behaviour such as breastfeeding, or smoking, but more challenging when developing, for example, a measure of public opinion that is both reliable (stable), and yet sufficiently sensitive to show change in response to an intervention.

Learning from experience

This brief overview of the issues in developing valid and reliable methods of measurement in health promotion provides a clear indication of the complexity of this task. Developing questions or a scale that will serve as the basis for the evaluation of program outcomes is not something that can be taken lightly. Often, practitioners will need to seek external advice from people with relevant research experience (see Box 5.1).

Although there are no comprehensive 'toolkits' for outcome measurement, much has been learned through careful experimentation in the past decades, and there is a growing range of standard methods for measuring health behaviours and determinants of health behaviours. For example, common definitions and survey instruments for measuring children's health behaviour have been established through a WHO-supported European cross-national research group (Aaro & Wold, 1989; Currie, 1994).

Similar attention to detail has been applied to the development of instruments that measure changes in the determinants of health behaviour, and in environmental factors. For example, in the past two decades considerable effort has been placed on developing tests and scales to develop valid and reliable measurements of personal and social determinants of behaviour, such as self-efficacy and social capital. Other studies have sought to evaluate environmental change, such as the introduction of restrictions on smoking in public places (Brownson et al., 2002).

The more consistent use of established measurement techniques, such as those referred to above, would not only do much to improve confidence in standards, but have the additional benefit of increasing comparability between studies.

> When planning an intervention, it is important to start the construction of an evaluation instrument by finding out what has been learned from the experience of others, and whether a 'standard' form of the measurement exists, which could be used or adapted to local or specific needs.

Commonly used techniques in questionnaire design

Questionnaires are the most commonly used measurement tool in health promotion. Questionnaires offer the opportunity to pose questions in a highly structured format, which invites responses within a carefully prescribed range, or in a less structured format, which allows a wider range of responses. The advantage of a structured format is knowing the measurement properties of an instrument, and in the level of control the researcher is able to exert over the issues covered and the detail of responses.

Closed questions ensure that each respondent considers the same issues such that results can be more easily compared, and summarised in numerical form. Against this, closed questions do not allow respondents to add information that they consider important in relation to the issues being addressed, and do not allow for qualification or explanation of responses, which may be essential in making sense of the information obtained. Figure 5.1 illustrates some of the different types of closed questions.

Open-ended questions have the opposite characteristics. They allow greater scope for explanation, qualification and improved understanding of issues. They often require qualitative analytic techniques, such as content and thematic analysis, and may provide rich information regarding the relevance of a health promotion intervention from the perspective of the individual. Against this, open questions often lead to inconsistent and unpredictable responses, they are more cumbersome to manage, and they require more effort to summarise. They provide useful contextual information that usually assists process, rather than outcome, evaluation.

The choice of format (or combination of question types) will depend upon the subject matter and the nature of the research. For example, if you are seeking people's opinions on new issues, or want to assess their understanding of issues, the use of open questions may be appropriate. If you want to assess behaviours or health-related practices within a limited range among organisations or individuals, closed questions may be more appropriate. Combining both formats is a particularly attractive option in many cases. These techniques of question construction and questionnaire design are considered in much greater detail in specialist texts on the subject, and again, where a previously established instrument is not available, it is worth obtaining more specialist advice on the development of appropriate survey instruments.

Measurement error and its consequences

Measurement error is the difference between the observed score (the actual measurement you have) and the true score on the phenomenon of interest. Measurement error can greatly reduce the possibility

There are several different types of closed question format that can be applied to elicit answers to different types of question. For some questions, a simple *yes/no* answer is all that is required. This is a *nominal* level of measurement. There is no ranking or order in the responses—they are simply labelled categories of response. For example:

Were you born in Australia?   Yes/No

In some cases, a *cumulative scale* (often known as a Guttman scale) may be used where it can be assumed that reaching one level in a hierarchy means that other levels have also been achieved. For example, in assessing educational achievement:

What is the highest level of education you have achieved? Tick one box:

Primary school ☐
High school ☐
Undergraduate degree ☐
Post-graduate degree ☐

In other cases, particularly in trying to assess people's attitudes towards an issue, a *Likert scale* can be used to assess degrees of agreement/acceptability of different propositions. These are ordered so that responses may range from one view or opinion to the opposite view or opinion about an issue or in response to a statement. For example:

How did you feel about going to school? Tick one box:

I liked school very much ☐
I liked school a little ☐
I didn't care one way or another ☐
I didn't like school much ☐
I didn't like school at all ☐

Other techniques for asking questions include *multiple choice*. This is commonly used to test knowledge of an issue by presenting a series of factual statements, some of which are correct and some not. Respondents have to identify the correct statements. *Rank ordering* of beliefs or preferences from different options may also be used in some circumstances to help indicate personal and collective priorities. Questions here would ask people to rank statements against each other. For example:

'Which are the most important areas of chronic disease prevention?' Rank these from 1, the most important, to 6, the least important:

_____ obesity prevention
_____ tobacco control
_____ injury prevention
_____ preventing illicit drug use
_____ sun protection
_____ blood pressure control

Screening and routing: Not all questions need to be answered by everyone. In many circumstances, it is appropriate to use a screenng question and to route those respondents who do not need to answer certain questions to the next stage of the questionnaire. For example:

Have you ever had your blood pressure measured?

Yes ☐
No ☐

Depending on the response, the subject can then be routed through the questionnaire. For example:

If no, go to question ...

If yes, answer the following question:

When did you last have your blood pressure measured? _____

Figure 5.1 Commonly used formats in closed question design

of finding a statistical effect or difference between intervention and control groups following the successful implementation of a health promotion program. This can lead to one of two types of incorrect conclusion: **type 1 error** or **type 2 error**.

A type 1 error is where the researcher concludes that a health promotion program has produced significant outcomes (positive or negative) when it has not. A type 2 error is where a program effect is said to be non-significant when in fact it is. Poor quality measurements can produce both types of error. A type 2 error may also occur when the study has low statistical power, with too few people in the study to detect the effects being sought, usually because the *sample size* was insufficient to detect the expected effect.

A hypothetical time-series design evaluation is shown in Figure 5.2. The figure shows the mean outcome score for two different measures of self-confidence that were used to assess the effects of an intervention to improve the confidence and skills of young people to refuse an offer of a cigarette from a peer. This illustrates the effects of measurement error, and also shows the idea of measurement reliability and responsiveness to an intervention.

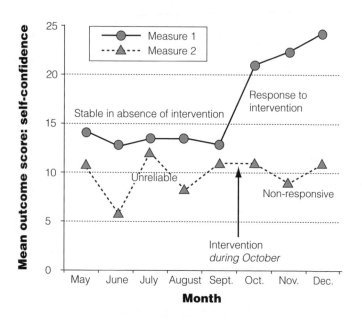

Figure 5.2 Reliability (reproducibility) and responsiveness of measurement: self-confidence

Measure 1 (the solid line) is stable (*reliable*) during serial administrations over the months May to September, with the mean scores being very similar. This indicates that the measure is stable and reproducible, as the outcome does not change in the absence of an intervention. The mean self-confidence score ranges around a value of 13–14. When the intervention in October occurs, the self-confidence score shows *responsiveness*, increasing to a value of 21 and continuing to increase to a score of 24 by December.

By contrast, measure 2 (the dotted line) has poor measurement properties for two reasons. It shows great variability preintervention, it is unstable, and not reliable, and then fails to show any responsiveness to the intervention. Hence, this measure will show possible effects in the absence of an intervention due to random variation, and will fail to show an effect if exposed to an intervention (both type 1 and type 2 errors referred to above), and hence its use may lead to the wrong conclusion regarding program effects.

Other errors and biases in the response to a measurement that can influence health promotion program evaluations include:

- *Response bias as a consequence of being observed*. People often report socially desirable answers to sensitive issues, such as substance use, sexual behaviours or domestic violence. Even the mode of administration of a questionnaire can influence the measurements observed. For example, adolescents will respond differently to questions about illicit drug use if asked in a deidentified school-completed questionnaire compared to household or telephone interviews. These biases can be reduced and managed by ensuring that questions are presented in a neutral form, and by reminding the subject that there is no 'right answer'. Ensuring confidentiality in the administration of the questionnaire and, whenever practical, offering anonymity to the subject will also help to reduce this source of bias.

- *Response bias as a consequence of sensitisation to the issue*. This is particularly a problem when the same questions are used on repeat occasions. This may result in a subject becoming curious about an issue, and might influence people in a control group to take action that they might not otherwise have taken. For example, if a person who smokes is asked in some detail about their smoking habit on several occasions, this in itself might prompt him or her to attempt to quit. This bias can be minimised by undertaking *cross-sectional* surveys of different subjects before and after an intervention, rather than conducting surveys with the same *cohort*. However, this may reduce the *statistical power* of the study (see Chapter 4).

- *Response changes as a consequence of the maturation of a group or cohort*. For example, longitudinal studies of adolescents over several years may show changes in attitudes or beliefs as a consequence of growing up, and changes in experience and physical maturation, which may be due to these ageing processes and not due to an intervention. Similarly, following older adults may show declines in some measures such as cognitive or functional status as a consequence of ageing, which may attenuate any positive intervention effect. These changes are not necessarily a source of error or bias, but need to be considered in the analysis of change over time in a cohort. In the same way, changes to the composition of communities over time may mean that serial cross-sectional survey samples from the same geographical area differ in sociodemographic attributes. If serial surveys are used to evaluate programs, then efforts to adjust for these differences are required.

It is almost impossible to remove all sources of error and bias from a health promotion evaluation. In most interventions involving communities or other population groups, there are simply too many elements that are beyond the reasonable control of a researcher. As a researcher, it is important to be aware of the major sources of error and bias, to do all that is possible to minimise their effect on a study, and to acknowledge the potential for error and bias in the discussion of results from a study. As a practitioner, it is important to be aware of potential error and bias when critically assessing the quality of a health promotion program evaluation.

Different measures for different purposes

Each stage in the planning and evaluation process may require different measures, and pose different measurement challenges. For example, in program planning and design, routinely collected information on mortality, morbidity and health behaviours might be used to determine the size and importance of issues that might become a priority for intervention. In the development of a health promotion intervention, formative evaluation measures may be used to assess the acceptability and potential reach of a program in a target population. In assessing the quality of the implementation, measures of participation, and of program quality, can be used.

The measurement of health promotion outcomes is one of the more challenging tasks, as reliable and valid measures are not routinely available and need to be developed or adapted for the specific purposes of the program. Longer term health outcome measurement can often be achieved through the use of existing measures, and sometimes through the use of routinely available health data. Beyond assessment of the effectiveness of a program (stage 4 of Figure 2.1), evaluation of the quality of dissemination requires measures of spread or diffusion of the programs into communities. These measures (such as uptake and acceptability) may be similar to the measures or indicators used in process evaluation.

Table 5.2 describes the different measurement and evaluation tasks, and provides examples of program measures for the different stages and phases in planning and evaluation.

Future challenges in measurement in health promotion

Health promotion has evolved from an individual focus on measures of knowledge, skills and behaviour through to a more complex set of group and organisation-level activities that require measures of social and physical environments and communities. This shift in focus requires a broader set of measures and variables to complement individually based measures. Similarly, in the consideration of interventions, a broad range of measures is required, not only to assess the impact of programs, but also to measure the process and health promotion outcomes.

> The challenge in health promotion measurement is to develop relevant indicators that meet the measurement needs for which they were intended, while at the same time collecting reliable information.

Table 5.3 shows an expanded framework for health promotion measures, across the different stages in the planning and evaluation

Table 5.2 Measurement in program evaluation

Stage of program and measurement needs	Examples of measures	Measurement and evaluation tasks
Program planning and design: formative evaluation	Responses of target group to testing of messages or program materials; perception of stakeholders of program's likely success	Sufficient sample size and sample variation to assess generalisability of formative findings
Program implementation: process measures; implementation indicators	Number or proportion of people attending program; number or percentage of professionals participating; program delivered as intended; environmental changes carried out as planned; interagency partnerships developed as planned	Reliability and validity of process measures; measurement properties of indicators, such as audits of program attendance, satisfaction measures, community partnership measures
Health promotion outcomes: individual level	Awareness of health issues; cognitive changes such as self-efficacy, intention to be more active, beliefs	Psychometric properties and construct validation of cognitive measures, social support and social capital measures; test–retest repeatability
Supra-individual measures	Social supports; enhanced social influences; social environment; social capital (collective efficacy)	Construct validation as above
Intermediate health outcomes (impact)	Behavioural changes; define general behaviours; are there specific domains of measurement?	Measurement properties, including criterion validity; are measurement domains part of same construct?
Physical environmental measures	Changes made to physical environments completed	Validity of environmental measures; inter-rater agreement using audit tools, objective environmental measures
Community-level change	Policies developed; program elements institutionalised in the (health or other) system; program elements self-sustaining	Reliability of policy measures; replication of process and impact effects
Long-term health outcomes	Reduced morbidity, or reduced disease incidence; improved wellbeing/quality of life	Validity of health outcomes or quality of life measures; predictive validity of intervention exposure on outcomes
Diffusion and dissemination of program	Spread of effective program and resultant policy—process evaluation of dissemination	Measures of dissemination and diffusion; uptake of program as proportion of eligible sites

Table 5.3 Typology of health promotion measures

Health promotion area	Concepts	Hypothetical examples of measures (variables)
Problem definition	Sociodemographic and geographic measures; measures of place or location; measures of community need; prevalence of health understanding, beliefs and behaviours	Socioeconomic status; measures of poverty or food insecurity; prevalence of high-risk sun exposure behaviours
Health promotion actions	Process evaluation measures; quality assurance measures	Measures of community development; sense of partnership in a community, or stakeholder-perceived degree of affiliation within a coalition
Health promotion outcomes	Individual-level measures: cognitive; affective	Knowledge, perceptions, beliefs, confidence, self-efficacy, resilience, behavioural intentions
	Social norms, social connections, empowerment	Measures of peer influence, social supports, social capital (social capital could be operationalised as an individual, social or community-level measure)
	Organisational, community and environmental-level measures	Measures of school climate; community capacity; physical environment measures—measures of urban form
Intermediate health promotion outcomes	Health behaviours; policy and environmental changes	Binge drinking rates; passive smoking exposure; changes in policies towards immunisation; changes in food supply policy
Health states or social conditions	Changes in disease incidence, complications or severity; changes in societal-level outcomes	Reduced incidence of diabetes; improved quality of life or functional status among cancer or stroke patients; improved community wellbeing

cycle described in Chapter 1—from 'problem definition' to 'outcomes assessment'. The middle column shows the 'concept' that is meant, and the right-hand column provides examples of variables, which operationalise the concept as a real measurement.

As indicated above, this task is challenging where there are no existing measures of the concept from which to learn. Where established measures exist, it is important to consider using them; the tasks of developing a new measure, understanding its measurement properties and refining it for use in interventions are substantial and resource intensive.

Much of the existing measurement development work has provided information regarding health beliefs, behaviours and other individual-level variables. The challenge for measurement specialists in health promotion is to develop better measures of the less tangible concepts required for health promotion evaluation. Clear and consistent definitions are required for concepts such as 'social capital', 'community empowerment' and the attributes of coalitions and partnerships. Existing measures are available for defining some problems, for individual-level health promotion and intermediate (impact) outcomes, and for health states. By contrast, few measures are available for health promotion actions, organisational or environmental outcomes, or community-level social outcomes.

To understand the nature of this challenge, consider the measurement needs in the evaluation of substance use prevention programs, immunisation trials or health promotion programs to reduce falls in the elderly. There are established measures of the behaviours of interest (use of alcohol, illicit drugs, being immunised, incident falls) and of attitudes and beliefs towards these issues (e.g. parents' views of the need for their child to be immunised). Risk factors for these behaviours have been described and are measurable (e.g. risks for injurious falls in the elderly). In the actual interventions, less attention may be focused on developing process measures, which may have important consequences if the program was not successful; lack of explanatory or implementation measurements may make it difficult to establish why a program did not work.

Environment-level measures are increasingly collected in injury programs, but may not have been collected in an immunisation program, where factors such as access or cost made it more difficult for parents to have their child immunised. The interorganisational partnerships required for comprehensive substance use or injury prevention programs (such as those needed between health, social welfare and educational agencies) may not have been established, or may not be functioning well; measures of these phenomena would inform the evaluation process. The endpoints of social and health outcomes are the least well conceptualised and measured. These are important outcome measures, especially in substance use prevention programs (e.g. individual and community-level measures of social capital, community crime rates or sense of coherence).

Summary

The primary goals of health promotion measurement are to assess health promotion phenomena accurately, and contribute to the best scientific evidence for assessing intervention effects. This chapter has provided an introduction to the wide range of different tasks and skills required to develop reliable, valid and responsive measures that can be used in the evaluation of health promotion interventions.

Measurement is important across all stages of program development and evaluation. In the health sciences, much research has occurred in quantifying the measurement properties, reliability and validity of observable phenomena. Health promotion program evaluations often require reliable and valid assessments of non-observable and 'subjective' phenomena, and assessing their change in response to interventions, and their role in explaining outcomes. This is a challenging task. To help understand measurement development in health promotion, this chapter provides examples of the wide range of methods used to develop reliable and valid measures in health promotion, and the statistical methods that will be encountered in measurement studies. As we have emphasised, the purpose here is for readers to become familiar with the names of these statistical tests and understand the context and purposes for which the test is used.

Although there are no comprehensive 'toolkits' for health promotion measurement, much has been learned in the past decades, and there is a growing range of standard methods for measuring health behaviours and determinants of health behaviours. The more consistent use of established measurement development techniques would not only do much to improve confidence in standards, but also have the additional benefit of increasing comparability among studies. When planning an intervention it is important to start the construction of an evaluation instrument by finding out what has been learned from the experience of others, and whether a 'standard' form of the measurement exists, which could be used or adapted to local or specific needs.

Health promotion has evolved from an individual focus on measures of knowledge, skills and behaviour through to a more complex set of group and organisation-level activities that require measures of social and physical environments and communities. This shift in focus requires for a broader set of measures and variables to complement individually based measures. Multiple disciplines, from urban planning and social ecology through to individual-level psychometric measures, will need to be explored in the evaluation of the next generation of health promotion programs. Only with broad disciplinary origins are we likely to develop rigorous and relevant measures of health promotion concepts, and assess whether these concepts are influenced by theoretically grounded health promotion programs.

References

Aaro, L.E., Wold, B. (1989), *Health Behaviour in Schoolchildren: A WHO Cross-National Survey: Research Protocol*, WHO (EURO), Copenhagen.

Ademiluyia, G., Rees, C., Sheard, C.E. (2003), 'Evaluating the Reliability and Validity of Three Tools to Assess the Quality of Health Information on the Internet', *Patient Education and Counseling*, 50, pp. 151–5.

Barrett, L.L., Plotnikoff, R.C., Raine, K., Anderson, D. (2005), 'Development of Measures of Organizational Leadership for Health Promotion', *Health Education and Behavior*, 32(2), pp. 195–207.

Brown, W., Trost, S., Bauman, A., Mummery, K., Owen, N. (2004), 'Test Retest Reliability of Four Physical Activity Measures Used in Populations', *Journal of Sports Medicine Science*, 7(2), pp. 205–15.

Brownson, R.C., Hopkins, D.P., Wakefield, M.A. (2002), 'Effects of Smoking Restrictions in the Workplace', *Annual Review of Public Health*, 23, pp. 333–48.

Currie, C. (1994), *Health and Health Behaviour Among Schoolchildren: A WHO Cross-National Study (HBSC) International Report*, WHO (EURO), Copenhagen.

de Guia, N.A., Cohen, J.E., Ashley, M.J., Ferrence, R., Rehm, J., Studlar, D.T. et al. (2003), 'Dimensions Underlying Legislator Support for Tobacco Control Policies', *Tobacco Control*, 12, pp. 133–9.

Further reading

Streiner, D.L., Norman, G.R. (2003), *Health Measurement Scales: A Practical Guide to Their Development and Use*, Oxford University Press, New York.

Chapter 6
Evidence, practice and the critical practitioner

Critical appraisal of research and evaluation evidence

One purpose of *Evaluation in a Nutshell* is to equip the reader with the ability to understand, interpret and assess the quality of published work in evaluation reports and in scientific journal papers. The preceding chapters have provided an introduction to many of the strategic and technical issues that arise in designing an evaluation, and some of the practical and scientific challenges that have to be addressed in executing the evaluation of a health promotion program. Recognising and understanding this broad range of issues will improve your ability to make judgments about the quality and relevance of 'evidence' from published research.

This ability to critically appraise the work of others is an important skill for all practitioners, researchers and decision makers. It enables us to read and interpret published reports, and make better judgments and decisions about the likely success of individual programs. *Critical appraisal* in health promotion can be done in a systematic way but, given the complexities in health promotion, requires a broad approach to judging the worth of interventions.

Box 6.1 (adapted from Bauman & Rissel, 2003) provides a critical appraisal framework that works as a checklist through which the health promotion relevance, as well as the methodological rigour, of a published study can be appraised. Clear quality criteria for formative, process and impact evaluation are described, and the importance of each of these elements can be considered in the context of each study.

Box 6.1 Critical appraisal of health promotion programs

Part A: appraisal of individual interventions

1. *Problem definition*
   - Is the health problem a health promotion priority?
   - What is the magnitude of the problem or its amenability to change (through an intervention)?
   - What is the overall purpose or goal of the intervention?

2. *Formative evaluation and program development*
   - Is there evidence of developmental work or piloting of the intervention or its component parts?
   - Was the final version of the intervention tested with people similar to the target group?
   - Is there an underlying theoretical framework or conceptual model for the intervention?
   - Are the intervention strategies and settings identified?

3. *Process evaluation*
   - Is there evidence of any process evaluation to monitor the implementation of the program components?
   - How many people received (attended or participated in) the intervention? Were they typical of the target group at large (or were they different from those who did not participate)?
   - Is there evidence that the program was well received by the target population?
   - Of all those who could participate or be included, how many actually did so?

4. *Research methods to appraise the stages of impact and outcome evaluation*
   General:
   - Is the target or intervention group clearly identified?
   - Is the timeframe for the proposed change clearly stated? Is it realistic?
   - Is there other corroborating evidence of the observed effects (either from changes in other outcomes or from qualitative evaluation data)?
   - What was the study (research) design used in this evaluation?

- Was it the best or most feasible study design that might have been used in this setting in this program evaluation within available resources?

Study sample:
- What is the source population who are the intervention participants (sample enrolled in the intervention)?
- Was the study sample(s) representative of the target population or were they a 'convenient' sample?
- What were the *selection effects* that might influence (bias) this study (e.g. non-representative sample of the target group)?

Measurement:
- Are there specified and measurable intervention objectives?
- Are all relevant outcomes assessed? How important are any omitted outcomes?
- Were the measuring tools reliable and valid, and were their measurement characteristics provided or cited?

Analysis:
- Was the sample size of participants in the study (i.e. the statistical power of the study) sufficient to detect any potential effects that might result from the intervention?
- Were there any factors that were not measured that might have influenced the findings?
- Were any of these extraneous influencing factors controlled for in the statistical analysis?
- Were the most appropriate approaches to analysis used?

5. *Interpretation of the results/discussion*
- Were the conclusions drawn by the author(s) justified by the data?
- Were the findings generalisable to the whole community or to similar populations/settings?
- Were significant effects of practical health promotion significance or were they simply of statistical significance?
- Did the formative or process evaluation components of the evaluation enable us to understand the health

promotion program better? Were these evaluation components omitted? Especially for negative studies, might additional information have been informative here?

- Is there a need for replication research in this area? If the intervention was ineffective, what other approaches might be developed to address this problem?

Part B: post-intervention appraisal—does it make a public health difference?

6. *Replication*
   - Has the initial effective intervention been trialled in other settings?
   - Were those settings diverse enough to indicate the population generalisability of this kind of intervention?
   - Were the programs implemented and delivered successfully (mostly adhering to program objectives and methods) in these different settings?
   - Are the results communicated to policy makers and to professionals and practitioners? Is there a defined advocacy strategy to communicate these results?

7. *Dissemination*
   - What mechanisms for dissemination are developed or suggested? What might be possible?
   - Is there evidence of changes by policy makers or professionals to support dissemination efforts?
   - What is the extent of dissemination and is it sufficient for *population reach*?
   - Are sufficient resources diverted to support the dissemination process?

8. *Institutionalisation*
   - Are there policy changes in place to support and resource an effective program?
   - Are there monitoring systems in place to assess program sustainability and quality control of the intervention?
   - Are there surveillance systems to monitor the outcome of interest at the population level (e.g. rates

of smoking in pregnancy, immunisation rates in preschoolers, new HIV positive seroconversions per year)?

Part C: systematic reviews and research synthesis— summarising the evidence across studies

9. *Types of systematic review*
   • non-systematic (or selective) review
   • planned systematic review
   • formal approach to pooling estimates from multiple studies (using statistical techniques of meta-analysis)

It follows that there are no absolute 'correct' answers for all forms of evaluation study. For example, for a local pilot program, emphasis might be placed on excellence in formative and process evaluation. For judging excellence in effectiveness studies, the standard criteria for assessing 'scientific' quality are used—evaluation design, measurement, sample size, and appropriate approaches to the analyses of the results (shown in stage 4 in Box 6.1). 'Critical appraisal' is about consideration of all aspects of a program *in context*.

This checklist could be used for reading any published evaluation, in a journal, report or monograph format. Starting with the problem definition, the schema here includes careful documentation of elements of formative and process evaluation (stages 2 and 3 in Box 6.1), as well as describing and assessing research methods following the principles of research design, measurement and minimising biases discussed in earlier chapters. By the time the discussion of the published paper is reached, an attempt should be made to assess the practice-based relevance and generalisability of the findings, and whether the evaluation comprehensively covered all the components of good program evaluation.

Criteria for the searching for the later phases of evaluation are shown in Part B of the checklist (stages 6–8 in Box 6.1). For example, you might be searching for replication studies or evidence of successful dissemination of a project prior to considering the local adoption of a program. A search for replication studies may include the '*grey literature*', which comprises government-led evaluations, published technical reports or monographs, or other documents. Many of these evaluation reports from public sector or not-for-profit agencies are available through the Internet.

Finally, Part C of the checklist provides guidelines for summarising the quality of different types of evidence reviews that are available for a defined content area. There are often electronic databases in which papers from public health and other disciplines are stored (such as Medline) and web-based compilations of evidence regarding the effectiveness of health promoting interventions (such as the Cochrane Collaboration health promotion reviews). Web links to these sources are provided in the references at the end of this chapter.

Strategies to optimise searches are important in reviewing an area of intervention (Part C of Box 6.1). Sometimes, researchers compile summaries of research in a field. This can be a haphazard accumulation of the papers encountered by a researcher, or a more systematic review following logical search rules and the use of judicious and relevant keywords. Reviews are more 'systematic' if clear research questions are identified, a search strategy is defined, and a comprehensive review of relevant databases is undertaken.

If outcomes are very similar or identical in measurement, and research designs are similar, then a quantitative pooled analysis can summarise the net effects of a particular kind of intervention. This is known as a *meta-analysis*, but is only possible where interventions and outcomes to be combined are very similar. In health promotion this is rare across studies, and so meta-analysis is less frequent than in clinical and biomedical research. Nonetheless, there are some formal health promotion meta-analyses, where most of the primary studies are controlled trials. Examples can be found through the Cochrane Collaboration on issues such as tobacco prevention trials for youth, smoking in pregnancy trials, and smoking cessation trials using various media, self-help materials or pharmacotherapy.

> The ability to find evidence by accessing relevant reported research, and the ability to critically appraise evidence, are core skills in health promotion.

These skills provide the platform for planning an intervention, and a basis for relevant evaluation design.

Getting evidence into practice

Improving the quality and effectiveness of health promotion interventions ultimately depends on our ability to use the evidence generated through research and evaluation to guide improvements in the practical interventions that have an impact on health and the quality of life—*getting research into practice*. In the Introduction we considered the diversity of perspectives to evaluation, noting that scientists, health practitioners, politicians and the wider community all have different views on what represents 'value' from a health promotion program, how success should be defined and what should be measured. It follows that defining what is 'effective' practice, 'best' practice or 'better' practice is, in part, a context-specific judgment.

Often, the research questions of greatest interest to public health practitioners, and the policy makers who make resources available, are often not the questions that the researchers were funded to answer. This means that decision makers and practitioners can often be frustrated in finding program evaluation information that is really useful to them. Solutions have to come from dialogue between researchers, practitioners and policy makers to improve the relevance of the research done, and make the findings from research and evaluation studies as relevant to practice as possible. Increasingly, the evaluations of health promotion programs are seen as multidisciplinary collaborations, with requirements for more timely and population-relevant outputs.

What will also be obvious from the preceding chapters is that it is very risky to make decisions about the effectiveness of programs based on the results of a single study. Replication and dissemination need to be carried out, tested and demonstrated for the elements of an effective program suitable for population change to be identified.

> Working out what components work, and which can be translated across different settings and social groups, remains a greater challenge than proving yet another individual-level program is effective.

Concluding comments: evaluation—art and science

A further major purpose of *Evaluation in a Nutshell* is to provide an introduction to technical issues in evaluation, and some of the challenges related to the evaluation of health promotion programs. What becomes clear from this introduction is that evaluating a health promotion intervention is both an art and a science.

The challenges we face stem from the diverse origins, goals and methods of health promotion programs. What should be clear from the preceding chapters is that evaluation should be integrated into a program plan from the beginning of an initial idea (and the formative research that supports it), through to widespread program dissemination that should lead to population health change. There are different evaluation designs and research methods required for these different stages of program development, implementation and dissemination.

The different needs of researchers and practitioners often result in the use of a range of qualitative and quantitative methods, producing 'evidence' for different purposes. Given this diversity, we need to make decisions regarding the extent, expenditure and methodological rigour required for a particular program evaluation. We work in an imperfect environment, and need to make the method fit the circumstances of the intervention. There is no single, correct evaluation design. Both qualitative and quantitative methods have an important place. Both can be done well and both done badly—one is not superior to the other.

For every health promotion intervention, careful formative and process evaluation are essential. Good program development and clear planning will ensure that a quality program is developed; careful monitoring of implementation will contribute to an understanding of why one program works and another does not. Process evaluation is often neglected, but it contributes to an understanding of the way the program worked that can inform subsequent program development and refinement. Process evaluation provides the foundation for subsequent evaluation of program effectiveness, and is the cornerstone of the evaluation of replication and dissemination of programs.

To evaluate the effectiveness of a program, especially when a program is being implemented for the first time, randomised controlled or quasi-experimental designs are the minimum standards for evaluation design. Established, reliable and valid impact measures should be used. The results should be assessed in terms of the observed *effect size*. Both qualitative and quantitative methods have an important place; together, they can provide different perspectives. This combination of perspectives can provide information on the acceptability and feasibility of interventions, as well as providing evidence of effectiveness.

Effective interventions need to be replicated in different settings to assess if they can be conducted and delivered to diverse populations. If replication shows the program is possible in other settings, then policy makers and practitioners need to be influenced to adopt and disseminate the program more widely. Only when an effective program is delivered across a whole region in a sustainable way can it produce a population-level health benefit.

Ultimately, not all of us have the opportunity or resources to undertake highly structured evaluation of our work. Better knowledge of the strategic and technical issues in health promotion evaluation not only enable us to make well-informed judgments of published work, but also enable us to better judge when, how and to what level we may need to evaluate our own work—as *critical practitioners*. This knowledge is also of great importance in managing the expectations of managers, program funders and the wider community.

References

Bauman, A, Rissel, C. (2003), 'Guidelines for Journal Reviewing', *Health Promotion Journal of Australia*, 14(2), pp. 79–82.

Cochrane Collaboration is available at http://www.cochrane.org. It produces and disseminates systematic reviews of healthcare interventions and promotes the search for evidence in the form of clinical trials and other studies of interventions. It provides a subscription-based, electronic research site providing access to these systematic reviews. There is also a Cochrane site dedicated to summarisng the effectiveness of health promotion and public health interventions: http://www.vichealth.vic. gov.au/cochrane/activities/reviews.htm.

Medline is available on the 'ISI Web of Knowledge' at http://isiknowldge. com, a subscription-based electronic research site providing access to high-quality information in the health and medical sciences (including Medline), social sciences, and arts and humanities, as well as search and analysis tools.

Further reading

Glasgow, R.E., Lichtenstein, E., Marcus, A.C. (2003),'Why Don't We See More Translation of Health Promotion Research to Practice? Rethinking the Efficacy-to-Effectiveness Transition', *American Journal of Public Health*, 93, pp. 1261–7.

Glossary[1]

Advocacy   the combination of actions designed to gain policy support, political commitment, and professional and community acceptance for a particular course of action to promote or enhance health

Behavioural epidemiology   the study of the distribution and determinants of behaviours that are related to health. It contributes to an understanding of the individual, social and environmental factors, and conditions that lead to health-enhancing or health-comprising behaviours

Bias   where something differs systematically from the true situation. Biases found in studies may be due to how people are selected for the study, the measurements used, or factors that may have influenced the observations made or associations found through analysis of data

Cluster randomised control trial   a randomised control trial (RCT) where randomisation occurs at the level of groups or communities. These groups or communities are randomly allocated to intervention or control conditions. This is necessary and appropriate where individuals within a community share features in common (are clustered), such as in worksites or school classes. See also *randomised controlled trial (RCT)*

Cohort   an identified group or population. In a cohort study, the same population is followed and assessed at each stage in the study, both before and after an intervention. A cohort is sometimes used in *quasi-experimental design* studies. See also *cross-sectional study*

Concept   an organising idea, often theoretical, used to describe a phenomenon that is not directly observable. In health promotion,

---

1   The definitions in this glossary are pragmatic definitions based on the authors' experiences in evaluation, research and practice in health promotion. More formal definitions can be found in publications such as J.M. Last (2000), *A Dictionary of Epidemiology*, Oxford University Press, Oxford, and D. Nutbeam (1999), 'Health Promotion Glossary', *Health Promotion International*, 13(4), pp. 349–64.

we use concepts such as community capacity, self-efficacy and social influence, and then try to develop operational measures of them. See also *observable phenomena*

Confidence interval   a statistical term used to describe the extent to which the true results are outside of a range of possible results described by the 'confidence limits' (the confidence limits or confidence interval includes a range of values within which the true value in the population is likely to lie)

Confounder   a variable that may influence the association between two other variables and thereby confound the results in a study. For example, a study may find that women have better preventive practices than men, indicating that gender is associated with preventive practices. However, another variable, not gender, may be causing this association. For example, women may have higher self-efficacy than men, and self-efficacy might be associated with preventive practices. Thus the relationship between gender and preventive practice may be due to differences in self-efficacy and not really due to gender itself. Here, self-efficacy is the confounder for the relationship between gender and preventive practice

Construct validity   see *validity*

Consultation   the process of engaging with or seeking the views of stakeholders or the community or target group members, with a view to enabling participation in intervention development, advocacy or policy formulation. See also *participatory planning*

Contamination   the amount to which control or comparison groups or communities are exposed to intervention elements. For example, in a community-wide campaign, the control communities may share some media channels in common with intervention communities. If they are exposed to the campaign messages, it will be more difficult to show greater program effects in the intervention community

Content validity   see *validity*

Correlate(s)   factors associated with other variables. For example, in a survey of teenagers, boys are more likely to be physically active than girls. It simply means that there is a statistical relationship between gender and physical activity. Correlation does not imply causality. See also *confounder* and *determinants*

Cross-sectional study   a survey or other form of data collection that is obtained at a single point in time from a population or population sample. Unlike in a *cohort* study, these individuals are not followed and assessed on a further occasion

Determinants   variables that 'cause' observed or measured outcomes. For example, cigarette smoking has been shown to 'cause' lung cancer through a series of steps that have established a clear and unequivocal relationship between smoking behaviour and subsequent risk of lung cancer. Establishing similar, unequivocal relationships between health promotion outcomes (such as knowledge or social attitudes) and subsequent behaviours is a continuing area of research endeavour. We often misuse the term 'determinants' when we really just mean that there is a statistical association between variables, or that they are *correlates*

Dissemination   an active and intentional process of achieving the maximum uptake of effective and feasible health promotion interventions into a community

Drop out or loss to follow up   the proportion of participants who start a program or are included in a study, and do not participate in follow-up activities or surveys—they are 'lost to follow up'. This may lead to *bias* in the results if those individuals who are followed up are systematically different from those not followed up. See also *non-response bias*

Effectiveness   the extent to which a health promotion intervention is successful in 'real-life' conditions in achieving the impact and outcomes that were predicted during the planning of the program

Efficacy   the extent to which a health promotion intervention is successful under controlled or 'best possible' conditions

Evaluation   the process of judging the value of something. In health promotion, an evaluation will determine the extent to which a program has achieved its desired outcomes, and will assess the different processes that led to these outcomes. Scientists, health practitioners, politicians and the wider community all have different views on what represents value from a health promotion program, how success should be defined and what should be measured. Hence, there is no 'correct approach' to health promotion evaluation; it is context specific. See also *formative evaluation, process evaluation* and *impact evaluation*

Evaluation design   the set of procedures and tasks that need to be carried out to examine the effects of a health promotion intervention. The purpose of a good evaluation design is to enable us to be as confident as possible that the health promotion intervention caused any changes that were observed

Face validity   see *validity*

Formative evaluation   a set of activities designed to develop and pretest program materials and methods. Formative evaluation occurs as part of program planning, and occurs before any elements of the program are implemented

Generalisable   the extent to which the findings from the study are likely to be reproduced in other groups or in the whole population. This is sometimes described as *external validity*

Goals   health promotion program goals are measurable changes in behaviours (e.g. smoking, food choices), or social, economic and environmental conditions (e.g. restrictions on smoking, food supply and promotion), which are the major determinants of the health outcomes (such as reduced heart disease or diabetes) that are being targeted. Program goals are an important intermediate outcome of health promotion programs

Health education any combination of educational resources, materials or educational methods that are designed to improve health-related knowledge, health literacy and increase skills that promote health

Health outcomes the long-term endpoints of a health promotion program. They may include reduced morbidity and mortality, improved quality of life and functional independence

Health promotion outcomes modifiable personal, social and environmental factors that are a means to changing the determinants of health (*intermediate health outcomes*). They also represent the more immediate results of planned health promotion activities

Impact evaluation a set of activities designed to assess short-term progress in the implementation of a health promotion intervention. This may include measurement of *health promotion outcomes*

Institutionalisation where a program has been successfully diffused into a community, has established policy support and funding mechanisms, and has continuing community support. At this stage, the program is integrated into the long-term functions of a host agency or organisation. This stage of evaluation is primarily concerned with quality control and long-term monitoring and surveillance of outcomes at a population level

Intermediate health outcomes the results of health promotion programs in the short term, which are measured by changes in lifestyle factors (e.g. food choices, physical activity, substance use), accessing preventive services or environment changes that are likely to lead to improved health outcomes

Internal consistency of a measurement assesses how well a group of items or questions 'hang together'. It assesses the consistency of results across items within a score or scale. It describes how well each question relates independently to the rest of the questions in a scale and how they relate overall

Level of measurement a way of describing *variables*. Levels of measurement range from continuous (interval) variables that can take an infinite number of values such as height or blood pressure. Ranked data has discrete categories of responses. Sometimes the data has only two categories (yes/no, smoker/non-smoker), which are described as 'dichotomous' variables

Likert scale a ranked form of a measurement where responders are asked to rate something on a scale (e.g. from 'strongly agree' to 'strongly disagree'); the scale has a bipolar nature (two ends of the scale are opposite views), and is presented in ranked order; there may be a middle point (e.g. 'neutral', or 'neither agree nor disagree'). Likert scales are typically 5-point scales

Logic model a way of describing the changes that the program is intended to bring about, defining what will happen during a program, in what order, and with what anticipated effects. This is a conceptual 'roadmap' or illustration of how the program elements might work. A logic model describes program inputs (human, financial and material resources), the context of the program (those factors that will influence the implementation and impact of the intervention) and describes the activities that make up the intervention (e.g. program events, groups, training, social marketing). In turn, these are linked to the levels of outcomes that these 'inputs' are expected to produce

Non-observable phenomena attributes or characteristics (such as knowledge, attitudes, public opinion, and even some health behaviours) that cannot be directly observed and measured and have to be indirectly assessed (e.g. through surveys that are self-completed, or questions asked though face-to-face or telephone interviews). See also *observable phenomena*

Non-response bias the differences in the variables of interest in a study between those participating or completing a study (or intervention program) and those who drop out or do not participate. The term 'subject retention' is a related idea; it refers to the difference in number of participants who start a program and those who actually complete it

Objectives health promotion program objectives are measurable changes to modifiable personal attributes (such as knowledge, motivations, skills), social norms and social support, and organisational factors (e.g. rules and processes) that influence the program goals. See also *health promotion outcomes*

Observable phenomena are attributes or characteristics that we want to measure that are directly observable. For example, height and weight, blood pressure or serum cholesterol levels can be assessed through direct measurement. See also *non-observable phenomena*

Outcome evaluation a set of activities designed to assess whether or not the program successfully achieved its *goals* (such as changes in health behaviours) and *objectives* (such as improved knowledge and skills). Usually, outcomes imply longer term changes such as health status, whereas shorter term endpoints are often described as program impact. See also *impact evaluation*

Participatory planning a process of engaging with communities or stakeholders to form partnerships. As a consequence of these partnerships, the program planning process is carried out through consultations and community fora to make decisions about the shape of programs, or changes that will impact on the community and improve health

Pilot testing a set of activities designed to assess the feasibility and/or relevance of intervention components (see *formative evaluation*). Pilot testing may also refer to measurement development and piloting of a measurement in a sample of people. This is used to assess the *reliability* and *validity* of the proposed measurement

Pre–post study   a one-group evaluation design (also known as a 'before–after study'). This is a relatively weak design with one group or population measured before and after an intervention. This design is often used in pilot studies to estimate the likely effect of an intervention, and is not recommended for use in the evaluation of innovative health promotion interventions

Prevalence   a measure that describes how many people are affected or have a particular problem in a defined population

Process evaluation   a set of activities designed to assess the success of program implementation. Process evaluation describes and explains what happens once the program has actually started, and the extent to which the program is implemented and delivered as planned

Program plan   usually a written document that specifies the interventions to be employed, the sequence of activities, the partnerships to be developed, the personnel to be involved at different stages and the costs of the interventions. See also *logic model*

Qualitative methods   descriptive and analytical research techniques that are used to explore and explain phenomena of interest. Methods include the use of focus groups (structured discussions with stakeholders or members of a target group), or directly learning from participating in or with target group members (ethnographic research or participant observation, sometimes called 'action research')

Quantitative methods   descriptive and analytic research techniques that are intended to produce numeric data amenable to statistical analysis. Such data allows statistical testing of comparisons between groups, trends over time or the strength of associations between variables

Quasi-experimental designs   evaluation designs that have defined control or comparison populations against which intervention group effects could be compared. The population or group receiving the intervention is predetermined and non-randomly assigned

Random sample   a *sample* drawn from a population where each individual has an equal probability of being chosen. Random sampling is intended to produce a sample of individuals that is representative of the population

Randomised controlled trial (RCT)   a research design where the individuals (or groups) receiving the intervention are not predetermined. Individuals or groups are randomly allocated to receive the program, or not to receive the program. Every individual or group has an equal chance of being offered the program, or not

Reach   a term used to describe the proportion of a target population that is engaged in the different elements of a health promotion intervention. Program reach is especially important in determining the generalisability of a program to a population as a whole. The concept of reach is also relevant to the *replication* and *dissemination* stages of program evaluation. See also *generalisable*

Reliability   the stability of a measure, assessing the extent to which each time the measure is used, and for each person it is used with, it will measure the same thing (give the same score or value). This is also referred to as 'test–retest reliability'. Another form of assessment of reliability is 'interrater reliability', which is where two individuals assess the same phenomenon and the level of agreement between them is described

Replication   the process of repeating an intervention in a different setting or with a different population or subgroup

Responsiveness   the capacity of a measurement for change in response to an intervention. The best responsive measures should show a substantial change following an intervention, but not change in the absence of an intervention

Sample   a group of individuals selected from a population for study, or to be the subjects for a health promotion intervention. See also *random sample*

Sample size calculation   how many people are needed for an evaluation study using standard statistical formulas. To do this, it is necessary to specify what quantitative change is expected or hoped for in the intervention (e.g. a 10% increase in breast cancer screening from 70–80% following the intervention).

Scales or scores   composite summaries of existing variables intended to produce an overall score to reflect an underlying dimension (e.g. six questions—or items—might be summed to produce an overall 'depression score')

Secular trends   the rate of background changes in a phenomenon in a population (e.g. national rates of smoking might be declining, and obesity may be increasing)

Social mobilisation   organised efforts to promote or enhance the actions and control of social groups over the determinants of health. This includes mobilisation of human and material resources in social action to overcome structural barriers to health, to enhance social support, and to reinforce social norms conducive to health

Statistical significance   a measure of the extent to which the relationship between variables, or observed results, from a study might have occurred by chance. Statistical significance is assessed after the application of appropriate statistical tests

Structured discussions   a qualitative research technique, the purpose of which is to elicit information or perceptions from structured questions that are defined in advance. Structured discussions may be with individuals, as semistructured interviews, or with groups of people, as in the conduct of focus groups

Time-series design   the set of procedures used to evaluate a health promotion intervention in which there are multiple measurements preceding intervention, followed by multiple post-intervention measurements of the outcome of interest

Triangulation   the process of comparing different evaluation findings that are accumulated from a variety of sources

Type 1 error   where the researcher concludes that a health promotion program has produced significant outcomes (positive or negative), when it has not. See also *type 2 error*

Type 2 error   where a program effect is said to be non-significant, when in fact it is. Poor quality measurements can produce both type 1 and type 2 errors. A type 2 error may also occur when the study is underpowered, with too few people in the study to detect the effects being sought, usually because the sample size was insufficient to detect the expected effect. See also *sample size calculation*

Validity   the assessment of the 'truth' of a measurement. A question, scale or test is considered valid to the extent it measures what it intended to measure. The concept of 'face validity' is that experts in the field think the measure is a useful way of assessing the dimension of interest. The concept of 'content validity' is that the items cover all of the potential areas of interest ('domains' of interest) expected for the measure. 'Construct validity' describes the extent to which the 'construct' that is being measured in a study (e.g. self-efficacy, social capital, or quality of life) is actually measured by the questions or items used in a study. The usual method for identifying a 'construct' is through statistical techniques, such as latent variable methods, exploratory or confirmatory factor analysis and internal consistency reliability, so that one can tell if the items seem statistically to be part of a single construct or dimension. This is known as 'construct validation'

Variables   quantitative measures that are (validly and reliably) assessed, and, as the name suggests, capable of showing variation between subjects, and variation in response to intervention. Variables may be single items (single questions), or summarised as composite *scales or scores*

Index